THE
REAPER'S DANCE

THE
REAPER'S DANCE

1000 DAYS OF COVID

Fourth Edition

Ravi R. Iyer, M.D.

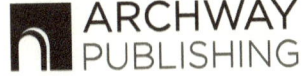

ARCHWAY PUBLISHING

Archway Publishing books may be ordered through booksellers or by contacting:

Archway Publishing
1663 Liberty Drive
Bloomington, IN 47403
www.archwaypublishing.com
844-669-3957

ISBN: 978-1-6657-4472-0 (sc)
ISBN: 978-1-6657-4471-3 (hc)
ISBN: 978-1-6657-4473-7 (e)

Library of Congress Control Number: 2023909697

Print information available on the last page.

Archway Publishing rev. date: 4/17/2024

CONTENTS

For my mother, who lit the lamp of self-expression in me,
For my father, who ignited the fire of resilience
and drove me to find myself,
For my wife, my steadfast champion,
For my children, who give meaning to it all,
For my staff, who support me in my purpose,
And most of all,
For my patients, who believed I could keep them safe.

To the many physicians, scientists, and patients whose personal stories of courage, folly, suffering, and hope were the inspiration for this book and the story it tells, in the hope that we may never again return to the horror of those dark days—the world owes all of you an immense debt of gratitude.

FOREWORD

A crucial election loomed in the Indian state of West Bengal in April 2021. Living in Singapore, my brother and I watched TV news with foreboding as India's Prime Minister Narendra Modi, ignoring the warnings of epidemiologists, addressed packed election rallies with tens of thousands of people in attendance, while the Delta variant ran amuck in a wave of disease and devastation. News and social media were awash with reports of hospitals turning patients away due to a lack of beds and of patients dying in hospitals that had run out of oxygen. Crematoria fires burned non-stop as the bodies piled up.

My parents lived in that state, and while they rarely ventured out, and always masked up when they did, I worried that the vector of the election rally-fueled infection would inevitably catch up with them.

A week later, despite receiving the 2nd dose of the Astra-Zeneca CoviShield vaccine both my parents were stricken with fever and the classic signs of the disease. Ironically they had caught the disease while waiting to be vaccinated in the overcrowded vaccination center!

I was in Singapore, behind closed borders and shutdown airlines. My parents were alone in Kolkata and the Reaper was standing by their bed! And so began my mother's 2-week battle with the Delta variant while my Dad was more fortunate with a milder version of the illness. As I frantically worked the phones to get a hospital bed for mom, I was acutely aware of the good fortune that provided me access to a network of resources that few could enjoy. One element was my cousin, Dr. Ravi Iyer, who had been on the frontlines of Covid for a year, in Virginia USA.

Chapter 9 of The Reaper's Dance speaks of the collaborative work of the GWAPI physicians as a consultative resource with Indian medical teams and my mother and I were direct recipients of this phenomenal network of courage and support that spanned the world. Together with other physicians, Dr. Iyer formed an informal medical advisory committee to support my family. When mum's condition worsened, he was there to strategize with me as to what I should request of the Indian doctor while simultaneously checking in with my father who was isolated at home. Both my parents recovered and the Reaper was denied his quarry.

In this book, Dr. Iyer has distilled a lifetime of experience in medical practice and research, as a frontline medical worker in the war against the Covid pandemic. He expands on the lab leak theory as well as the hypothesis that the SARS-CoV2 virus jumped from animals to humans at the Wuhan wet market; he explains the mechanism by which the virus infects the human body, and how mutations occur; he shines a light on the policy and communication missteps of the Trump administration, and the fog of disinformation that frontline medical workers had to encounter.

And he shows a mirror to all of us. He compels us to examine our role in the global cycle of consumption, how we infuse our own biases with a sense of righteousness that reduces our ability to reach across the aisle in discourse and to lend a helping hand to others.

With continuing destruction of habitats bringing humans into close contact with wild animals, the probability of a new virus making a similar jump from animals to humans is a very real possibility. We must learn lessons from the Covid pandemic if we are to stand a better chance at saving lives and preventing mass economic distress to millions.

Informed and enlightened voters are the most powerful way to hold elected officials to account and make decisions that build our long-term capacity to tackle a health emergency. In an engaging narrative style, The Reaper's Dance empowers us to understand the mechanisms that led to the spread of the Covid-19 pandemic. It makes an urgent case to address gaps in healthcare systems and infrastructure, and to respect the science.

The next time around, we can do better. We must do better.

Anusha Bhagat

INTRODUCTION

To say that the COVID-19 pandemic shook the world is like saying the eruption of Mt. Vesuvius of Pompei was a wakeup call. In every way the pandemic with its immediate threat to life and survival as well as the chaos of the response to it completely shattered the human psyche across the globe. The idea for this book evolved slowly over 2020 and 2021 out of my team's experiences here at The Iyer Clinic on the frontlines of healthcare during the pandemic. The work we did at the clinic very quickly impressed on me the overpowering need to educate the public about serious issues facing them. I could see that my forty years as a physician was directly undermined by multiple forces that were destroying the fabric of human interconnectedness, and that leaders and public health authorities were doing an abysmal job in communicating the lessons that needed to be taught. The human experience is multifaceted and complex. It would be a grave injustice to cast everyone into a single dimensional story. There is no single hero or villain in this story and even the most egregious offender did do some things wonderfully well, while some of the greatest champions in the public health arena had their feet mired in some pretty dark dirt. When humans are brought face to face with their own fragile mortality and look into the abysmal blackness of the eye sockets of death, the veneer of pretentious morality is stripped bare, and the true substance of their character becomes revealed. The pandemic laid bare the human psyche at its most elemental level and for an intense 18-month period human society came to grips with existential questions of what it means to be human and have a relationship with us and our fellows. In this 2nd

edition of The Reaper's Dance, I take you, the reader, by hand through the days, weeks, and months of the journey we walked at the clinic and elsewhere while unraveling the story of the pandemic piece by piece for you to see, experience and absorb. Unlike other works the story of the Covid pandemic is still evolving and new information regarding its origins is emerging almost daily and lending urgency to the need for comprehensive reforms in the way we oversee and regulate all such research. Most of all this book is a plea and a pathway to understanding the essential interconnectedness that we have to each other and the health of even a blade of grass on every continent of this fragile planet.

CHAPTER 1

The Gathering Storm

At the end of time, when the many become one, the last storm shall gather its angry winds to destroy a land already dying. And at its center, the blind man shall stand upon his own grave. There he shall see again, and weep for what has been wrought.

—Robert Jordan, *The Prophecies of the Dragon, the Essanik Cycle.*

The Beginning

Thursday February 27, 2020

Mr. Hutchinson got out of his car at the Dulles Town Center mall. His faithful Labrador dog was turning eight years old that weekend. He was excited. He loved that dog. *Eight years!* he thought as he walked toward the pet superstore. *It's been quite a journey. A new kennel would make a perfect gift.* He walked into the mall, crossing a line of window displays. He stopped and window-shopped a bit. A group of tourists bustled past him chattering excitedly as he strolled along gazing at the window displays. He walked into the pet store, stopping to pick up some treats for Oscar from a side aisle. The options were many, but he finally found a salesperson who was able to help, and he stood in line at the checkout counter with a kennel that was the perfect size for his dog.

Pushing his cart with the large kennel out of the store, Hutchinson felt a little shaky. He glanced at his watch. It was half past noon, and he hadn't had any breakfast. Even though he had not taken his diabetic medications that morning, Hutchinson knew the telltale signs of low sugar. He had better eat. He rolled the cart toward the food court in the mall center, stopping at a Dunkin Donuts shop to pick up a frosted doughnut. He sat down at a table in the food court. The doughnut was a taste of sugar heaven. The crowd of shoppers passed his table, chattering excitedly as they stood in line at the Chinese food stall. *Tourists*, thought Hutchinson as he bit into his doughnut.

Behind him. a couple coughed loudly and then sneezed.

Hutchinson turned slightly.

"Excuse me," the woman said, smiling apologetically.

Hutchinson smiled and nodded an acknowledgment. His doughnut was finished anyway, and he felt stronger. He got up to leave.

***

Saturday February 29, 2020

Hutchinson woke up feeling woozy. There was a dull headache, and his head felt heavy, like a hangover. He walked into the bathroom, reached into the cabinet, and popped a couple of pills of Tylenol. The party the previous day must have been too much, he thought, making a mental note to turn in early that night. He walked down to the kitchen to pop a Keurig coffee pod into the machine. The sound of coffee percolating into his cup filled the kitchen. But this time, the accompanying aroma was absent. He picked up the cup and sipped as he reached for his iPhone. *Strange*, he thought. *The coffee tastes funny.*

He turned toward the back door as a wave of dizziness washed over him. He staggered in midstride, and then, steadying himself, he walked out into the yard to breathe the cool morning air. He was breathing harder than usual. Oscar came bounding out of his new kennel, and

Hutchinson stepped forward to greet him. His heart was hammering, and the ground suddenly appeared to tilt. He wondered why Oscar was looking down at him.

Wow. He must have grown, he thought.

But then, why were the trees in the sky? Across the backyard, Mrs. Clarke, watched from her house as Mr. Hutchinson, her neighbor, appeared to stagger and then fall. Oscar was licking his face. Mrs. Clarke screamed his name multiple times, but he didn't respond. Panic-stricken, she dialed 9-1-1.

A Predictable Life

March 1, 2020

I pulled off the highway from Atlanta to Vienna, Virginia, for a pit stop at a highway gas station. In the back of my Honda Pilot, my German shepherd was restive, sensing an opportunity to jump out and relieve himself. Little did I realize as I walked over to the restroom of the gas station that, in another week, I would no longer take for granted the simple freedom of brushing elbows with unknown crowds or stand in proximity to them at the checkout counter. On the other side of the US continent, in the western coastal city of Seattle, someone I knew nothing about had gasped out their last breath. In another ten days, the rippling echo of that gasp would rip apart all our lives in a tsunami of fear, disease, death, and disinformation. But my happy ignorance of the looming maelstrom would afford me a few more days of bliss, and I continued my drive home from training at South Metro Atlanta Schutzhund Club.[1] Tomorrow, it would be life as usual at the medical clinic I ran in Herndon, Virginia.

For twenty-three years, the Iyer Clinic had been a focal point for primary care and adult general medicine for northern Virginia's

---

[1] Mike DeFabo, "Schutzhund: A Sport for Working Dogs." *Times West Virginian*, October 17, 2013, https://www.timeswv.com/sports/schutzhund-a-sport-for-working-dogs/article_1906ddf4-0386-53cc-9d01-bd81a9b88450.html

exploding population. Located in western Fairfax County, the clinic served all of Fairfax and Loudoun County, two of the wealthiest counties in the United States with an ethnically diverse and highly educated population. Northern Virginia, with its concentration of federal, information technology, and biopharmaceutical industries clustered around the seat of the most powerful government in the world, has an incredible concentration of knowledge workers. Patients in this community have the resources to obtain care and the education to understand the mechanisms of disease. But as the course of events over the next two years would show, this intellectual capacity would put them at a special disadvantage when faced with the volume of disinformation that would assail them.

On March 1, 2020, the Sunday edition of The New York Times would announce, that President Trump's statements dismissing the public's fears as the U.S. reported its first death from COVID.[2] And none of my doctor colleagues or my staff had any real concern that our lives would change in any way. The 2020 presidential election cycle had just begun, and the United States was in the grip of an unusually polarized public debate. White America was in the throes of an identity crisis. Black America was discovering its voice. And immigrant America was struggling for admittance to the American dream and for acceptance, assimilation, and recognition. Politicians on both sides of the aisle were beating their favorite drums, pitching the beats that were most in synch with the pulse of their constituents.

The phenomenon of the COVID-19 pandemic in the United States is as much a story of the evolution of American consciousness and the way science, media, and the body politic would handle the dissemination of facts and information as it is a story of the virus and the disease it wrought. A perspective piece by Mary Bassett and Natalia Linos in the March 2, 2020, Washington Post warned that the dangers of the institutional mistrust, rejection of science, anti-immigration policies,

---

[2] Michael Crowley, Mike Baker, and Nicholas Bogel-Burroughs, "Trump Moves to Calm Fears as First U.S. Death from Coronavirus Is Reported," *New York Times*, March 1, 2020, A28.

the penchant for alternative facts as narratives in the political and public domain along with growing social and economic inequities make the current climate in the U.S. ripe for catastrophe.[3]

A Leaf from History

March 4, 2020

A memo from the administration of Stone Springs Hospital Center in Aldie, Virginia popped up in my inbox, alerting me that the hospital was closing the open walkway between the multispecialty suite in the physician's office building and the main hospital to exert access control of patient traffic through predefined portals of entry that could be regulated for infection control. The move would not affect the operations of The Iyer Clinic Stone Springs office, but it was a sign that times were changing.

Concerned by the growing rumbles of an impending health-care crisis, I contacted my liaison with Sunrise Laboratories to ensure the clinic had the supplies necessary to perform RT-PCR tests for COVID. I was assured we would be well stocked, which, by itself, was rather exceptional for any laboratory at that time since very few locations had any testing capability in those days. The critical problem was not the ability to do the test but, rather, the ability to collect the nasal samples containing the infective virus. The specimen collection and viral transport medium used in the testing process was in global short supply.

March 10, 2020

At the clinic. we were still operating in a bubble of secure confidence. The virus was a news item, but we had seen other outbreaks and had

---

[3] Mary T. Basset, MD, MPH, is the director of the FXB Center for Health and Human Rights, Harvard University. Natalia Linos MSc., ScD, is a social epidemiologist and executive director of the FXB Center for Health and Human Rights, Harvard University.

never so much as seen a single case. During the H1N1 epidemic of 2009, I had seen only a few cases of serious illness. The Ebola outbreak of 2014–2016, which had spread to the United States, had produced a scare. And even though I was interviewed about it on ABC news, we did not have any alteration in our daily routines and never saw a single case. Still, in my community of friends in northern Virginia, as well as my friends in the Schutzhund sport community, I was getting an increasing number of concerned enquiries about the virus and the disease it caused.

I reassured everyone this was not likely to become serious, but then an article in The Washington Post caught my eye. It was an analysis by Dali L. Yang, a professor of political science at the University of Chicago who specialized in research on governance and regulation in China. [4] Yang wrote about critical missteps by the authorities in Wuhan with a combination of political interference, hubris, and bureaucratic meddling between December 31, 2019, and January 20, 2020. This interference ensured that frontline whistleblowers in the medical community who raised alarm about a new respiratory illness they were seeing were dismissed, censured, or otherwise silenced. In addition, the criteria for a diagnosis of viral pneumonia of unknown etiology (VPUE) were made so stringent by the Wuhan Health Commission that it was virtually impossible in those early days to diagnose even a single case as caused by a coronavirus. This response by the Chinese of obfuscation, deflection, denial, and censorship was typical of their management strategy and had been seen earlier in the first SARS-CoV-1 outbreak of 2003.[5] The Dali Yang article impressed upon me that things could well be no different this time around.

I clicked open a tab on my Chrome browser to my Amazon account and immediately placed an order for four 3M partial face mask respirators with filter cartridges, ten boxes of BioSafe Face shields, several

---

[4] Dali L. Yang, "Wuhan Officials Tried to Cover up COVID-19—and Sent It Careening Outward," *The Washington Post*, March 10, 2020.

[5] A. Ahmad, R. Krumkamp, and R. Reintjes, "Controlling SARS: A review on China's Response Compared with other SARS-affected Countries," *Trop Med Int Health* Suppl 1 (November 2009): 36–45, doi: 10.1111/j.1365-3156.2008.02146.x, epub June 5, 2009, PMID: 19508440, PMCID: PMC7169812.

cases of Nitrile gloves, and one gallon of concentrated swimming pool disinfectant. It would be sixteen months before I would be able to order any of those items again.

My next order was placed on Alibaba.com for two PAPRs (powered air purifying respirators) units for $450 each. These purchases would prove incredibly prescient for my staff and my patients. Indeed, in all of Loudoun Medical Group of three hundred providers, we would be the only community clinic with total personal protection of a level of sophistication that would rival what was available in the best hospital ICUs of the nation.

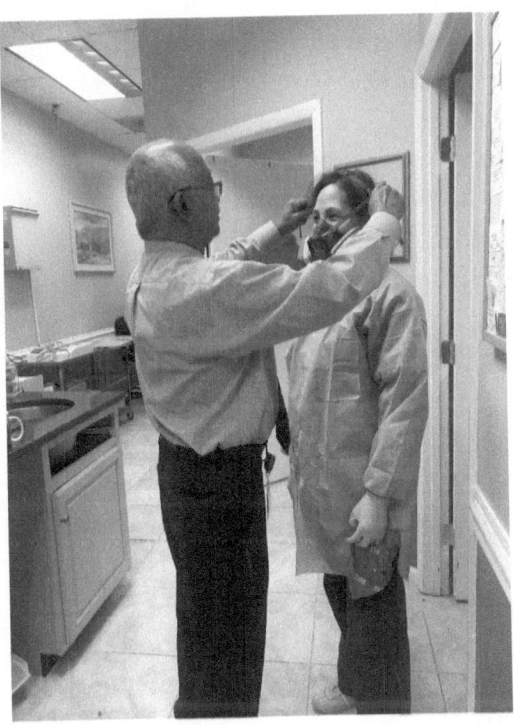

A Global Pandemic

On March 11, 2020, the WHO declared COVID-19 a global pandemic, and the US government began its hesitant and conflicted approach to its public health policy. The ability of a virus to spread in a population can be classified on three levels—(1) endemic, (2) epidemic, and (3) pandemic.[6]

Endemic disease is when the virus is restricted to few geographical regions; this restriction is due to a unique combination of environment and presence of a mix of immune and susceptible (nonimmune) individuals that produces local natural reservoirs for the virus to multiply and that restricts the disease to that area. The rates of disease prevalence and spread are predictable in an endemic area.

Epidemic is defined by the CDC as an "unexpected increase in the number of disease cases in a geographical area."[7] Terms like "outbreak" carry the same meaning as epidemic but apply to smaller geographical areas. A "cluster" is a collection of cases grouped into a single location like a home or a housing complex or residential community.

By contrast, a "pandemic" is defined as when the growth of disease cases is exponential, with the number of cases each day being greater than the day prior and spreading to several countries, often with skip areas in between, implying that the disease is jumping across multinational borders.

The formal announcement of the pandemic was received with conflicting responses at the clinic. At this moment in the trajectory of the pandemic, very little was known about the virus except that it was a respiratory virus spread by airborne droplets. None of us knew how long the virus survived outside the body. Questions were asked like, "Can you catch it by touching someone?" and "What if I touch a doorknob or some other mundane object?"

A telling example is of the Princess Cruise line story. In February 2020, a Princess Cruise line ship docked in Japan with seven hundred COVID-positive passengers, three of whom would later die. After the

---

[6] Columbia Mailman School of Public Health, "Epidemic, Endemic, Pandemic: What are the Differences?" Global Health, Infectious Disease, Public Health Education, February 19, 2021, https://www.publichealth.columbia.edu/public-health-now/news/epidemic-endemic-pandemic-what-are-differences.

[7] CDC, "Lesson 1: Introduction to Epidemiology," https://www.cdc.gov/csels/dsepd/ss1978/lesson1/section11.html.

passengers were off-loaded into quarantine, the cruise line advertised a worldwide search for sophisticated environmental disinfections and cleaning service provider who would have to abide by standards laid out by the Japanese Ministry of Health, the US Centers for Disease Control and Prevention, the World Health Organization, and the cruise line.[8]

Since there was no SARS-CoV-2-specific knowledge at that time, disinfection policy manuals were being written based on sanitation policies designed for gastrointestinal viruses like norovirus, which have very long survival rates outside the body on surfaces. When asked, experts hemmed and hawed, but the truth was no one knew and, even worse, no one had the courage to be honest about their ignorance. From the president of the United States down to the lowest CDC functionary, not a single individual authoritatively said, "We do not know." In the absence of definitive knowledge and with every "expert" on various media channels pontificating on their recipe during their fifteen minutes of fame, these standards were being concocted on the fly. These would then percolate worldwide through the public consciousness as fact. The stage was being set for speculative supposition to be paraded as established science.

Fight, Flight, Freeze, or Faint

When there is no definite answer, all answers are equally probable. And the default response of the population worldwide, therefore, was either one of overwhelming fear and caution or outright denial and whistle-in-graveyard bravado. Public health agencies at that time were proposing mandatory two-week quarantines not only for infected patients but also for all known contacts. My staff were obviously worried. Would we have to close the clinic down if an infected person walked in?

So, when I declared on March 12 that the Iyer Clinic would not

---

[8] Hannah Sampson, "Cruises Know How to Clean after an Illness Outbreak. But What Does a Coronavirus Cleanup Look Like?" **Washington Post**, February 28, 2020.

turn away any patient with respiratory or flu-like illness, I was met with fear and trepidation from staff and physician colleagues alike. Even my friends and family stood up against this decision, declaring that I was being foolish and needlessly exposing myself and others to risk. My wife, Anu, had her ears filled with these fears and opinions. And even though I was confident, I would be less than human if I too had not been at least somewhat troubled by doubts about my safety.

To her credit Anu simply said, "Ravi knows what to do and how to do his work."

Privately, though, she too did worry that something bad may happen to me. My career in research had equipped me with expertise in handling dangerous microorganisms safely, but I was soon to realize that most physicians lacked basic microbiological handling skills. Concepts like management of the burden of exposure to a pathogen before an infection can happen were foreign to them. For the majority, at that moment in the evolution of the SARS-CoV-2 pandemic, the response was that they would get infected if they happened to simply be in the vicinity of an infected person. My argument that I knew how to manage risk against pathogenic exposure was not convincing to everyone around me. I, on the other hand, felt profoundly frustrated by the lack of true infectious epidemiology experience among my professional colleagues. To my staff, I said, "We are healers. We are the last line that stands between disease and death for the people who come to our door. If we are overwhelmed by fear than what is the purpose of everything we have done for 40 years? If we run or close our doors then what are we? This we can never do! The Iyer Clinic will never close its doors and we will find a way to remain safe and remain open and keep our patients safe."

In those early days of gloom and doom, trained physicians opted to shutter their practice without any rational insight into how to conduct themselves safely in the presence of a novel respiratory virus or take steps to acquire the skills necessary to keep their operations running. Physician groups were panicking. Several took out small business disaster loans or tapped into the federal Payroll Protection Program. The level of anxiety and fear was astronomical among private physician practices. Practices scrambled to reorient and realign their interests with large health-care players in the belief that their survival would be assured under a larger umbrella. Groups that struggled looked upon practices that remained open and thrived with significant angst and hostility. For the first six to nine months of the pandemic, the degree of hostility between physician practices was incredible, and in certain cases, petty retribution was exerted between practices in this competitive shark-fest of panic-ridden survival.

At our clinic, my two physician colleagues and I were able to remain focused on our mission through the fear-ridden atmosphere, as our patient volumes surged, and we continued to perform and thrive. We were not totally immune to being worried about our own safety, but all three of us shared a deep conviction in our duty to our patients, and this would sustain us in the darkest of times.

Most physicians who closed their practices during lockdowns did not expect the pandemic to continue for as long as it did. They assumed that things would reopen in thirty to sixty days. When practices closed their doors, their patients began to seek out other avenues of health care. Practices that remained open saw a surge in volume of two to three times their previous caseload. When practices that shuttered finally realized it would be months or even years before life returned to a semblance of normal, it was too late. They had lost their patients and their staff to other health providers who remained open.

The pandemic created very sharp divides between haves and have-nots, between those with knowledge and those without, and between those who were adaptable and those who were rigid. And these divisions were not temporary loss calculations with the opportunity to live to win another day. It was existence or extinction, with no second chances.

First Encounter

March 13, 2020

My phone beeped out an incoming text alert. It was from a patient. His wife and he were burning up with fever, and both had lost their sense of smell and taste. They would be the first COVID patients of our clinic over the next two years—the first of about fifty thousand COVID tests we would administer and about five thousand COVID-positive patients we would treat. The reaper was pounding at the Iyer Clinic doors!

I asked my patients to show up in the parking lot and informed my staff that our first COVID patients would be coming in about thirty minutes. The reactions to this announcement were as if I had exploded a bomb. My staff was fearful. My physician colleagues were aghast and declared I was going to push the clinic into a state-mandated lockdown. When the patients arrived, I met them in their car in the parking lot dressed in white hazmat overalls.

The husband and wife were seated in the rear seat and chauffeured by their adult son. Both were burning up with fever and looked sick. They had that tired, glazed look of illness in their eyes. In the months that would follow, I would become an expert in recognizing what I would begin to call COVID facies. It was a peculiar combination of body and face appearance that would betray the presence of the virus almost as accurately as the RT-PCR test for COVID.

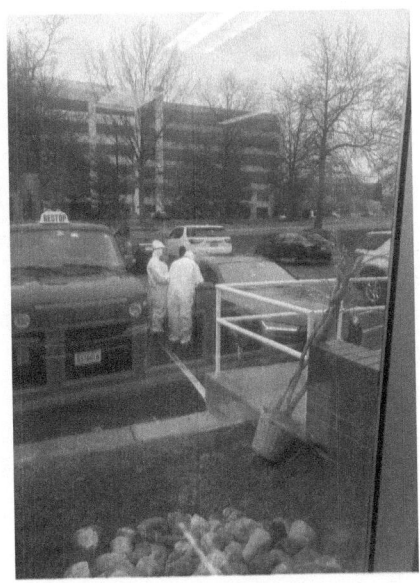

They were scared, and their eyes searched my face for reassurance. A quick check of their hearts, lungs, and vitals was optimistic. Their pulse oximetry was 99 percent saturation at room air, their lungs had good air movement to the bases, and both of their heart rates were fast but regular. I reassured them; gave them instructions on self-care; wrote out orders for vitamins, hydration, and supplements; and prepared to collect nasal samples for the virus.

While the entire clinic watched from behind glass windows, I quickly swabbed their noses and collected samples of nasal discharge into tubes of viral transport media. When I walked back into the clinic, people scurried away as if I was carrying the black death itself. Even the lab staff responsible for processing the sample and sending it to Sunrise Laboratories was nervous. People were washing their hands and almost bathing in sanitizer fluids. The level of hysteria was almost comical if it were not simultaneously tragic. I began to see how intensely contagious mass hysteria could become and how such pervasive fears could lead to ostracization or worse. At the back of my mind was a small niggling fear that my decisions may damage the clinic or, worse, the safety of my staff who depended on me.

A Shield against Evil

It was obvious to me that the only hope of overcoming this would be education and the power of example. The capacity of education to transform is immense. Decades prior to the pandemic, I had experienced the liberating power of education firsthand in my medical college in India. My medical college, despite being an excellent teaching school, unfortunately, was also dominated by rival student gangs that had overtaken the dorm environment.

This was no small matter. In my first day at medical school, I opened the door of my dorm-room to a knock and confronted a senior student who handed me a shoebox and asked me to stash it beneath my bed. When I asked what it contained, he said, "Country-made pipe bombs." He then went on to explain calmly that, since his name was on the police roster, his room could be subject to surprise searches.

I could hardly argue with a man who was holding a bunch of bombs, so I did as I was told. I slept over those bombs for a whole year and never cleaned the floor beneath my bed! I continued to study and focus on my career surrounded by the sounds of random gunfire, raucous drinking, and wild partying in the rooms adjacent to mine.

But fate was to take a hand in steering my life differently. A few months later, when exams rolled around, I happened to help one of the senior gangster students pass his exam by teaching him a few chapters of biochemistry. That student had been failing for several years, and so his passing was cause for incredulous celebration. Soon, the gang management decided that "Iyer" was too valuable a resource to be used to assist a single student at a time, so I was given a small room to conduct my tutoring classes for several students at a time.

Word spread about my classes and attendance grew. I was a second-year student, but I was reading up on subjects far above my level and explaining them to those who wished to learn. A small lamp of learning, a nucleus of something transformational had taken hold, and its effect was rapidly growing.

Even in those days I had an appreciation of having stumbled on something incredibly powerful—the transformative power of knowledge. I would study late into the night preparing for the next day's classes and relieve the intensity of study by taking walks at 3:00 a.m. in the darkness of the campus gardens, with the only light being the one streaming from my window.

My students began to do well in class, and word spread about the "Iyer classes." The decree went out among all gang members; "No one should touch Iyer!" Wherever I went, my status of privileged teacher was as good as bulletproof armor.

One day, two students from a rival faction came to the class. An uproar erupted between the faction controlling my dorm and the opposite group. Frustrated by the interference, I declared that my classes would be available to everyone, or they would be available to no one. Death threats and all manner of pressures were brought to bear, but I remained inflexible. After all, sleeping over bombs for a year does tend to instill a certain degree of bravado.

Eventually, a compromise was worked out, and I was allowed to teach all comers until two months before exams. After that, my classes would be available only to members of my dorm.

The episode taught me several things. First, if you have a valuable skill, then make it available to all who seek it without restriction. Second, if you truly have a valuable skill, then all the aces are in your hands. And if you understand how to allow everyone to win something, then you will be allowed to rule. I had discovered that knowledge is the ultimate equalizer and can overcome negativity and always create opportunity for freedom in all places. Little did I realize then how providence was preparing me for the pandemic that would come forty years later.

I began by first calling the staff at Sunrise Laboratories to the clinic for an in-service training session on how to safely collect nasal swab specimens for viral testing. Next, I focused on our staff. We had received an email from the chairman of our medical group alerting us to "start to plan for significant reductions in revenue." We were to manage this risk by actions that may include "staff furloughs, reduced employee hours and a reduction in provider compensation."

I laid out the scenario before my staff. "We have only two options before us," I told them. "We can close our doors to all sick patients. This will mean we will face furloughs and severe reductions in working hours and revenue but no real reduction in our risk for exposure to or for contracting the disease. All of us must still live and move in an outer world and among family members who can and will bring the disease to us. Or, the way I see it, the only way to handle this is to face it head-on. You cannot run, and you cannot hide. If you trust me to keep you safe, then I can show you how to conduct yourself and live so we can continue to remain fully open and functional, and all of you remain well through this crisis."

My staff voted to remain open. So began our transformation from a standard primary care clinic into northern Virginia's first and busiest community COVID testing and treatment center.

Facing the Enemy

We are not living in fear. We are living in faith.
—*Caring Bridge*

At the outset, we faced a unique problem. Our first two patients were still struggling with their recovery in isolation at home. They were being tended to by their college-aged son, who was still negative for COVID. The wife called us in a panic one morning. Her husband had passed out in the bathroom and fallen, hurting his wrist. What do I recommend? The question for us was what were we to do with those patients who were too sick to come to the office but not sick enough to go to the hospital?

The patient's wife was worried that, if he went to the hospital, he may be admitted. And in those days, the hospital was a riskier place to be than anywhere else. My staff, by now, was beginning to adopt my mission of creating a safe space free from fear. We got together. The nurses put together a mobile COVID provider kit, and we set off on what would become the first of many COVID house calls. We set up a pop-up camp portable shower privacy stall in the driveway of the patient's house and used it to change into our hazmat PPE and PAPR gear. We walked into the house dressed like astronauts in our moon suits with the neighbors watching from behind their windows in amazement at the tableau unfolding in front of them. It was like a scene out of the movie Outbreak.

My patients were isolated in separate bedrooms upstairs. I quickly examined the husband and determined there was no fracture, and he was simply dehydrated. Writing out an oral hydration recipe, I explained to the son an aggressive hydration regimen. Then we walked back out into the driveway; spray disinfected each other; and then de-gowned, discarding our PPE into large trash bags that we sealed and disposed, with an audience of the entire neighborhood watching us do our thing.

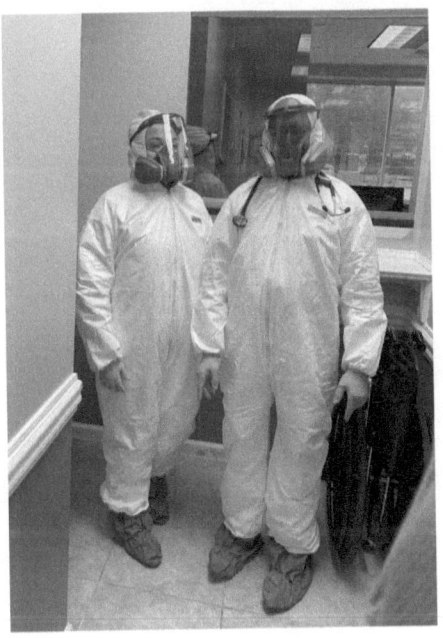

Looking back, it seems simple now. But then, it was something else. It was the first time we were translating our infection control and containment knowledge and strategies into real-world use in environments we did not have total control over. More importantly, at that point in the pandemic, what we were daring to do had not been done in community medical care, so it was incredibly new territory for all of us.

But the greatest impact was the experience of the patients themselves. The sheer relief in the patients' and their families' faces as we walked into their homes was something I will remember the rest of my days. It was as if some dark, menacing cloud had been lifted from their hearts. From our perspective, what we offered had no component of medication because no medicine existed. But in a world where no one could hug or touch or even come close to each other for fear of a lethal disease, at a time when even neighbors were shunning each other when sick, the fact that we were able to come into their home, acting and moving without fear of contagion and touching and examining them, had an incredibly powerful therapeutic effect. I had come face-to-face, hand-to-touch with the heart of health care — CARE!

CHAPTER 2

You Shall Not Pass!

I am a servant of the Secret Fire, wielder of the Flame of
Anor. The dark fire will not avail you, Flame of Udun!
Go back to the shadow. You Shall Not Pass!
　　　　　—Gandalf the Grey, Lord of the Rings:
　　　　　　　　　　The Fellowship of the Ring

The most important aspect of a physician's work is the creation of a safe space, a sanctuary where the patient can be free from fear of disease. Everything flows from this germinal aspect.

"Fear is the first contagion, not the virus. We must make ourselves, our presence, our clinic and wherever we are be a safe space for our patients." This was my insistent mantra at the office. Fear was a corrosive cancer that had to be addressed. It was ironic that, on one hand, we were focusing on eradicating fear in the community we served, and, on the other hand, we were surrounded by politicians, leaders, and media who knew of no language to speak other than fear and division. Indeed, the disinformation, fearmongering, finger-pointing, and divisive rhetoric of 2020 was, in many ways, more toxic than the SARS-CoV-2 virus itself. It was easier to handle the disease, as compared to the conversation in America.

When I diagnosed my first two patients on March 13 with COVID, I had very little to offer them other than supportive care, rest, lots of fluids, vitamin C, vitamin D, zinc supplements, and instruction to sleep twelve to fourteen hours per day. Neither vaccine nor antiviral treatment existed. But the one thing we had in plentiful supply was reassurance and, most important, 24-7 availability!

Nothing truly tests your capacity as a healer than to attempt to deliver health care with no other tools at your disposal than your personal presence and ability to connect with the ailing patient. Many years earlier when I was starting out as a physician, I was taught a lesson by my George Washington University residency program mentor, Dr. Stanley Talpers. A tall, patrician, old-school physician, Dr. Talpers was the kind of fatherly doctor who inspired respect on first sight. He would always impress upon me the importance of addressing what he called "the real problem." "The real problem, Dr. Iyer," he would say, "is not the disease you diagnose. It is the unasked, unspoken question in the patient's heart about how he or she is going to live from this moment forward. At all times, you must show the patient that you understand the real problem and that you will be able to enable him or her to successfully navigate it.

"The practice of medicine," he would insist, "is the ability of the physician to impress upon the patient that, from this moment forward, they are no longer alone in their fight. They have you as their steadfast champion. And it does not matter that you may have no medicine in your hands. From this moment on, they have you standing guard at their door as their advocate between them and death. And if you do your job well, even if you lose, know that death will stop first and seek your permission to step aside so it may claim the patient." Dr. Talpers' words would come back to memory many times during the pandemic.

On March 17, a French team of doctors published a report on the use of hydroxychloroquine in combination with azithromycin on twenty-nine hospitalized COVID patients, showing a reduction in viral load as measured by nasal swabs on day six of the treatment. [9] The paper set

---

[9] Philippe Gautret, Jean-Christophe Lagier, Philippe Parola, Van Thuan Hoang, Line Meddeb, Morgane Mailhe, Barbara Doudier, Johan Courjon, Valérie Giordanengo, Vera Esteves Vieira, Hervé Tissot Dupont, Stéphane Honoré, Philippe Colson, Eric Chabrière, Bernard La Scola, Jean-Marc Rolain, Philippe Brouqui, and Didier Raoult, "Hydroxychloroquine and Azithromycin as a

off a firestorm of excitement worldwide. In India, the Indian Council
of Medical Research (ICMR) published a bulletin recommending the
use of hydroxychloroquine for prophylaxis in asymptomatic health-
care workers caring for suspected or confirmed patients and household
contacts of confirmed patients.[10] Similar decisions were being taken by
policy institutions of countries across the world based on these early
presumptive data. China, African nations, Europe, Italy, and other
nations all explored the possible utility of hydroxychloroquine and other
existing drugs as a potential panacea for a virus few understood well at
that time.

President Trump, who had faced withering criticism over his
decisions in January 2020 to downplay the seriousness of the pandemic,
immediately seized on this as his Holy Grail of redemption, with
tweets extolling its virtues. The impact was gargantuan.[11] Patients
began clamoring for the drug, and even physicians began prescribing
it to their COVID patients. Between March 19, 2020, and May 20,
2020, nearly 50 percent of physicians in northern Virginia had written
hydroxychloroquine prescriptions for their patients. In India and Africa,
hydroxychloroquine was being dispensed by social workers to the general
population like peppermint. All of this stopped by June 2020, when it
was established that the drug had little value at best and significant risks
at worst.[12] But by then, the impact on the scientific dialogue about the

Treatment of COVID-19: Results of an Open-Label Non-Randomized Clinical
Trial," *International Journal of Antimicrobial Agents* 56, no. 1 (2020).

[10] National Task Force for COVID-19, "Advisory on the use of Hydroxychloroquine
as prophylaxis for SARS-CoV-2 infection," New Delhi: ICMR, March 22, 2020
(cited April 14, 2020), https://icmr.nic.in/sites/default/files/upload_documents/
HCQ_Recommendation_22March_final_MM_V2.pdf.

[11] K. Niburski and O. Niburski, "Impact of Trump's Promotion of Unproven
COVID-19 Treatments and Subsequent Internet Trends: Observational Study," *J
Med Internet Res* 22, no. 11 (November 20, 2020): e20044, doi: 10.2196/20044,
PMID: 33151895; PMCID: PMC7685699.

[12] M. D'Cruz, "The ICMR Bulletin on Targeted Hydroxychloroquine Prophylaxis
for COVID-19: Need to interpret with Caution," *Indian Journal of Medical Ethics*
5, no. 2 (April–June 2020): 100–102, DOI: 10.20529/ijme.2020.040, PMID:
32393448.

virus and its management and the public health policies surrounding the pandemic had already occurred.

Worldwide, this episode illustrated a major aspect of the pandemic. Just as jet travel eliminated physical distances and had facilitated the spread of the virus, the instant communication of the internet and the availability of Google to research all forms of knowledge made information disseminatable without the context of wisdom.

Lock Her Up!

March 2020

When Toby and his wife returned from the Make America Great Again (MAGA) rally, it was a lively day. Donald Trump had been on the floor, surrounded by tremendous positive energy and die-hard supporters. There had been chanting, roaring, and everything else! "Lock 'er up! Lock 'er up! Lock 'er up!" the crowd had chanted. The gathering had been powerful and passionate, and the presence of old and veteran Republicans had added to the excitement. Now, on arriving home, Toby had a sore throat. Must be from all that "Lock Her Up" chanting, he thought.

But it became worse. The next morning, he began coughing. His breath seemed on fire, and his head felt woozy. He could not smell or taste anything. His wife, Angelina, called her best friend Sybil:

Angelina. Hey, Sybil, I hope I am not bothering you at this time.

Sybil. No! Obviously no! What's the matter?

Angelina. Toby is continuously coughing, and he has a temperature! I'm worried! He'll be OK, right?

Sybil. Yes! Don't worry! My neighbor Mrs. Oliver has just shared with me an article about a miraculous drug for the China virus!

Angelina. Is Toby suffering from COVID!? Oh! No!

Sybil. Angelina, calm down! It is not confirmed yet. And I hope it is not a virus. But still, it's good to take a few measures.

Angelina. What does the article say? The coughing will stop, right?

Sybil. Yes! It's about hydroxychloroquine. Give Toby two tablets of it; you will see the difference! I have some that I got from my doctor. You can have some from me.

Angelina. Oh, Sybil You're an angel. How much should I give to Toby! Do you hear that? He's still coughing, and he's all the way in the other room!

Sybil. Yeah, I can. But don't worry, please! I read it in the article. It's the best medicine for the virus.

Angelina. I'll be right over.

Sybil. Sure! I'm here, Angelina. You take your time.

Later, Angelina went upstairs and gave Toby the medicine Sybil had shared with some warm water. She again checked his temperature; it was high, around 100 to 102 Fahrenheit. She rushed back to her phone:

Angelina. Hey, Sybil. Toby is still burning up!

Sybil. Relax! You've given him the medicine. Now he'll be fine.

Angelina. Do you know what's happening around? What is this new virus? Is COVID real? Trump seemed to have a different opinion in the rally.

Sybil. Yes. It's quite real People around us are suffering from it. It is bad, really bad. I was watching FOX news, and they're talking about having a global pandemic—a lockdown!

Angelina. What? A lockdown?! What does that mean? Is the virus spreading rapidly?

Sybil. Yes! It's all over the place now. Countries are going into hibernation for a while. There will be no jets in the air. I was shocked when I heard that a secret political mission was being carried out in the world. Bill Gates might be involved in all this. He wants to put a chip in all of us. Bloody virus!

Angelina. What chip? Bill Gates! Are you sure? How can an American do something like that to a fellow American?

Sybil. It's all international, Angelina. China has prepared this virus in the direction of some underground world mafia. God bless us all!

Angelina. Yeah, God bless us all. OK, I gotta go. I have to check on Toby.

Internet Experts

During the pandemic, everyone became an instant expert in all things without the requirement of either the apprenticeship or the discipline needed to command that knowledge. For the first time in the history of man, the drama of a worldwide disease was being played out in the arena of public consciousness and conversation, with absolutely no filters of discrimination or insight. Like the stream of consciousness speeches of Trumpian rallies, the media argued, promoted, and propounded every hypothesis, theory, and fact with equal weight. All of this produced intense disorientation of the lay public's sense of reality and stability. At a time when every breath was potentially toxic and common acts of human connection, a hug, a touch was all tainted with risk, people were experiencing intense isolation and distrust at physical, emotional, metaphysical, and psychological levels.

All this directly impacted on our work in the clinic as we tried to follow our mission statement of creating a safe space free of fear. Patients would pressure us with all kinds of literature pulled from the internet. Every article propounding the protective benefits of all manner of medicines was brought out for our opinion or analysis by patients eager to save their loved ones from the prospect of a lonely death in a hospital ICU. In our staff meetings we called this collective pressure upon us, from the disease besetting our patients, the risk to our own health, the ever-present fear of clinic closure, the polarized political rhetoric, the snake oil medicine promotion, the conspiracy theorists, as "the Balrog," naming it after the mythical horned, fire-breathing demon of the deep in The Lord of the Rings movie. We would end our meetings with the collective cry, "You shall not pass," echoing the famous words of opposition spoken by Ian McKellen, who played the character of Gandalf the Grey in the movie.[13]

---

[13] "I am a servant of the Secret Fire, wielder of the Flame of Anor. The dark fire will not avail you, Flame of Udun! Go back to the shadow. You Shall Not Pass!" Ian McKellen as Gandalf the Grey in Lord of the Rings: The Fellowship of the Ring.

The Frontliners

March 20, 2020

The first step I had to take was to change the physical workflow in the clinic. Together with my physician partners, who by now were firmly supportive of my plan, we changed our outgoing telephone scripts and began asking patients if they had any respiratory symptoms. If they did, they were told to wait in their cars and that we would come out and provide service at their vehicles. Next was airflow and ventilation control. My colleague tapped into his resource network and procured large plexiglass screens that were installed on the staff counters in the waiting room. In addition to plexiglass screens on patient facing check-in and checkout areas, we installed small fans that circulated airflow away from these areas. At the parking lot, we would clip on a small fan on the patient's car and hang a flexible transparent sheet over the car window such that we remained isolated from the patient as we worked with only our arms inside the vehicles space.

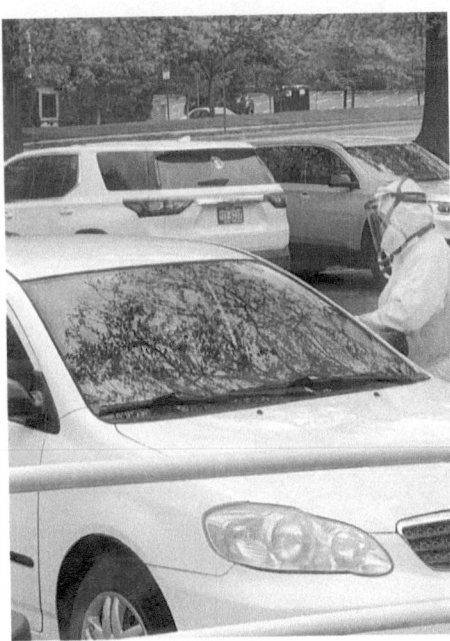

Inside the clinic we installed four UV air purifiers that constantly recirculated the air. We instituted a two-person work team operating in a buddy system. Two people would meet the patient in the car, and each would watch out for the other person's safety. We would constantly monitor each other for any unconscious break in our exposure, contact, or infection control protocol. An unconscious hand movement, a tear in a glove, an accidental contact with a nasal swab as we were withdrawing it and placing it into the sample container—any lapse was immediately handled with a spray of disinfectant on us by our partner. We adopted a habit of talking to patients with our hands clasped together like monks so we would not have any unconscious touch with the patient or with ourselves.

Even though I had a huge supply of disposable hazmat overalls, I soon realized we could ill afford to use disposable personal protection equipment (PPE) that was not really a reimbursable item by insurance companies. So, we switched to reusable, disinfect-able, whole-body polyester coveralls.

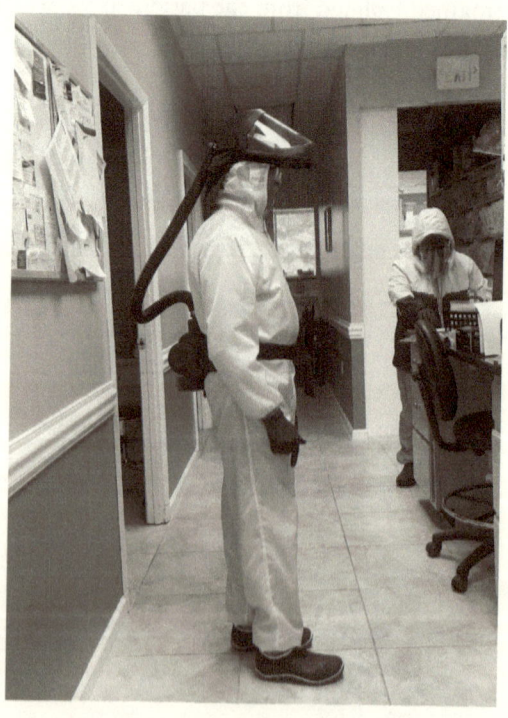

As a trained biochemist, I knew that silver, copper, and zinc ions are toxic to bacteria and viruses. An online search turned up a simple process I could use to develop a protocol for treating our PPE clothing such that they were impregnated with copper and zinc nanoparticles, increasing the level of protection we had while working with sick patients.[14] We used the same nanoparticle impregnation method to create copper-zinc-calcinated, turmeric-impregnated pre-filters that we inserted into the air intakes of our 3M respirators and the PAPR units, such that all the air we inspired reached our nostrils after passing through the most comprehensive viricidal filters we could create. Instead of expensive disposable paper booties covers, we switched to rubber garden shoes for everyone, which could be easily disinfected.

Everyone in the clinic would change into their work attire every morning and hang up their home clothing in a closet. At the end of the day, they would change back and go home.

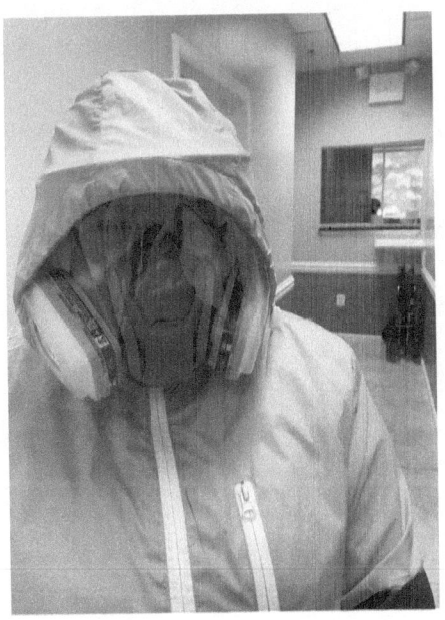

[14] Ali Sedighi, Majid Montazer, and Nahid Hemmatinejad, "Copper Nanoparticles on Bleached Cotton Fabric: In Situ Synthesis and Characterization," *Cellulose* 21 (2014): 2,119–2132, 10.1007/s10570-014-0215-5.

In a world where no one could get any medical-grade disposable gowns, there was a plentiful supply of colorful polyester hoodie windbreakers and snow pants that we purchased and distributed to all our staff. These were easily disinfected or cleaned in a washing machine's hot water cycle and reused. While Lysol and Clorox and bleach were unavailable, there was an abundant supply of swimming pool disinfectant concentrate by the gallon. A one-gallon jug of concentrated swimming pool disinfectant that we purchased in March 2020 was still in use at the clinic as of this writing thirty months later.

We hung our PPE in a closet equipped with a UVC light on a fifteen-minute timer. At the end of the day, we would switch on the light and expose our clothing to fifteen minutes of UVC irradiation. While we did use surgical masks in the clinic, I also promoted the use of face shields, since I knew that, unless you were using a fit-tested N95 mask, the protection of a face shield was equal to that of any loose-fitting surgical face mask and, from a social perspective, was superior since it allowed the emotional connection of visible facial features, which had a direct therapeutic benefit in health-care encounters.

At every step the mantra was "Adapt, Pivot, Connect, and Protect."

Tell It to the Stars

This trait of adaptability in any crisis and ability to retain control over the narratives of my life had had come to me at a very early age—by way of a powerfully moving lesson taught by my grandfather when I was in school. I was always popular enough in school and was gifted with enough intelligence to maintain decent grades, punctuated by flashes of excellence without too much effort. My successes in athletics contributed to my social status, and life was good. Then everything seemed to go wrong. A new teacher seemed to be out to destroy me in class. Some of my best friends moved to a different school. Overnight, I went from liking to hating going to school. I did not know what was wrong with what I was doing. Suddenly, whatever had worked before was no longer any good. Of course, I was sure I had nothing to do with this situation. It was that teacher; she hated me. It was all those other kids in class who would not include me. Amid this, my family decided to spend the weekend with my grandparents. That evening after dinner, my grandfather asked me if I would like to accompany him on his evening walk. I said yes, and so we set out.

After we'd gone a little distance, my grandfather asked me, "What's bothering you?"

"Nothing," I answered.

"Come on now," he said. "I know something is troubling you."

And then in a breathless rush, I unleashed my torrent of complaints.

My grandfather listened silently, and then when I stopped, he gently asked, "Are you finished?"

"Yes," I muttered sullenly.

"I want you to do me a favor," he said. "Do you see those stars?"

I looked at him, puzzled. The stars were bright against the velvety black curtain of the tropical night. "Yeah," I said.

He continued, "I want you to repeat all your problems to those stars—not in your mind but loudly. Speak out like the way you told me. Only this time, tell it to the stars!"

I looked at my grandfather, feeling confused and bewildered. The old man must be losing it, I thought. However, I dared not refuse. Sheepishly at first and then with growing confidence, I poured my litany of troubles to the vast and silent heavens. Finally, when I was done, I stopped and looked at him with a mixture of defiance, curiosity, and expectation.

There was a long pause as he gazed back into my eyes, and then he spoke, "Ravi, I now want you to look very carefully and tell me what the stars are doing with your problems."

"What do you mean, what they are doing?!" I exploded in irritation. "They are not going to do anything! Nobody can do anything! Nobody cares!"

He let the sound of my outburst die away before he answered softly, "Do you see now the benign indifference with which the universe regards your problems?"

I was stunned. With one soft-spoken sentence, my grandfather had rocked me out of my self-absorbed world of self-pity.

Then as the full impact of this shocking revelation descended upon me, he continued with immense gentleness. "Ravi, when the sun shines or when the rain falls, the sun is not shining to make the flowers bloom or to ripen the fruit. Neither does the sun shine to scorch the land and cause drought and famine. The rain does not fall to water the grass or to make the plants and trees grow. Neither does it fall to cause floods, death, and devastation. All the sun is doing is shining, and all the rain is doing is falling." He paused. "It is we who make a story out of it."

He looked down at me with a gentle smile. "Now, when it is you who makes the story, why do you want to make miserable stories?"

I looked at this old wise man who had just dynamited the bedrock of my self-assurance from beneath my feet. On that night, I saw that each one of us lives our lives with a lot of complaints. We begin compiling this list very early. As infants in the crib, we let loose full-throated protests over the delayed bottle of milk or the sticky wet feeling on our bottoms. Later, as we learn to compare, we always do so to our disadvantage. It is always the other kid or our brother or sister who got the better deal, the added advantage—not us. Still later, we extend this kind of analysis and judgment to our coworkers, superiors, and subordinates. Our complaints become a kind of yellow film that covers our eyes. leaving us with a jaundiced view of even the most fortunate circumstances that may befall us.

Decades had passed since that night with my grandpa under the stars, and now, faced with the pandemic of the century and the crisis of my lifetime, I saw very clearly the kind of story I needed to create. It was The Three Musketeers' motto — "All for one and one for all."[15] It was that and, "You shall not pass!"

---

[15] *Les Trois Mousquetaires* at Project Gutenberg, chapter 9: "Et maintenant, messieurs, dit d'Artagnan sans se donner la peine d'expliquer sa conduite à Porthos, tous pour un, un pour tous, c'est notre devise, n'est-ce pas?" (*The Three Musketeers* at Project Gutenberg, chapter 9: "And now, gentlemen," said d'Artagnan, without stopping to explain his conduct to Porthos, "All for one, one for all—that is our motto, is it not?")

CHAPTER 3

A Captainless Ship

A captain always knows where his ship is. It's like a psychic bond. If only we had a captain here.

—Marissa Meyer

A flock needs a shepherd, an army needs a general, and a ship needs its captain. If there was a single narrative about the story of COVID in the United States and the rest of the world, it was that of a ship without a captain. Nothing illustrates the damage done to the management of the pandemic more than the story of the masking guidance in the United States.[16]

Masks Are Unnecessary

In late February, 2020, the U S Surgeon General Dr. Jerome Adams, tweeted that wearing a face mask would not prevent the public from contracting the novel coronavirus. But strangely he insisted that the same ineffective masks would be essential for the protection of healthcare workers as they cared for sick people. The obvious contradictions in his logic was not lost upon the general public and only served to undermine

---

[16] Deborah Netburn, "A Timeline of the CDC's Advice on Face Masks," *Los Angeles Times*, July 27, 2021, https://www.latimes.com/science/story/2021-07-27/timeline-cdc-mask-guidance-during-covid-19-pandemic.

his credibility and the public's faith in the guidance being provided by the authorities.

By mid-March, businesses, schools, and restaurants were under mandatory lockdown orders in multiple US cities. Still the CDC's masking guidance on March 24, 2020, encouraged healthy people not engaged in healthcare or caring for a sick person to not wear masks. The COVID death rate and sickness statistics in the US at the time of this statement was 12,916 active cases and 1317 deaths.

Evidence grew by April that asymptomatic and minimally symptomatic people were spreading the virus during the first three- to five-day prodromal period after infection, prompting federal health officials to change their guidance after insisting for weeks to the contrary, to urge people aged two or older to mask up in public places and around high risk individuals.

By mid-July 2020, Dr. Robert Redfield, director of CDC, was urging everyone to wear masks and going so far as to forecast bringing the pandemic under control within two months if everyone wore a mask. The push to wear masks by everyone at all places and make it mandatory in air travel, government buildings, health-care facilities, and public transportation continued for the rest of 2020 and through February 2021.

But while this push was being advocated by public health authorities, President Trump, along with a majority of MAGA Republicans, publicly flouted masking by personal example, creating huge conflicts in public behavior. Just a few days after recovering from his own COVID infection, Trump tweeted his now infamous flu tweet. [17]

Not only did Trump's tweet misrepresent the toll of annual flu deaths, it also dismissed the COVID-19 death toll (approximately 5,400 daily deaths) as "normal." His rhetorical question, "Are we going to close down our country [for the flu]?" inaccurately conflated the mortality risk

---

[17] @realDonaldTrump. "Flu season is coming up! Many people every year, sometimes over 100,000, and despite the Vaccine, die from the Flu. Are we going to close down our Country? No, we have learned to live with it, just like we are learning to live with Covid, in most populations far less lethal!!!"

of seasonal flu with that of COVID, implying it was not worth changing collective behavior for such a low risk. Trump's flawed comparison directly exhorted people to not take the spread of the virus seriously.

At the Iyer Clinic, not a day passed without an encounter with an irate, maskless patient who challenged our polite request to wear a mask while within the clinic. While most patients were polite and considerate of public health and clinic policies, some of the altercations with rebellious patients bordered on physical violence, and all this would add to the constant stress of the pandemic.

Then on March 8, 2021, the CDC relaxed mandatory masking guidance for fully vaccinated individuals. There followed a five-month period of relaxed masking guidelines, only to be replaced, on July 27, 2021, with a return to full masking indoors in response to the Delta variant surge.[18] This continued through the remainder of 2021 and into summer 2022, when both masking and social distancing requirements were essentially made optional.

Get Protected, Wear a Mask

Janice pulled her car into the parking lot in front of her place of work. A thirty-eight-year-old single mother with two children, Janice could not afford to miss a day of work. I have no PTO, Janice thought. At least my job is essential and not shut down by this pandemic. She reached into her handbag to pull out a pink face mask. It smelled of yesterday's stale makeup.

I must get this washed, she thought. This year has been crazy!

She really hated the stifling feeling of the mask. Her breath felt hot and heavy as it moved through the fabric. Last year, she would never have believed her life would be like this. Everything was in short supply.

[18] Jing Huang, Brian T. Fisher, Vicky Tam, Zi Wang, Lihai Song, Jiasheng Shi, Caroline La Rochelle, Xi Wang, Jeffrey S. Morris, Susan E. Coffin, and David M. Rubin, "The Effectiveness of Government Masking Mandates on COVID-19 County-Level Case Incidence across the United States," *Health Affairs* 41, no.3 (March 2022): 445–53.

There were no paper towels, no toilet paper, no hand sanitizer; even liquid detergent was becoming hard to find. On top of it, this damn mask! She pushed the door open and walked down the corridor to her desk where she worked as a receptionist in a doctor's office.

She readjusted the cloth mask. It feels claustrophobic. That's what it is, she thought. And my glasses keep fogging up. She pulled the mask down until it was barely touching the tip of her nose. It was more comfortable that way. Last week, a memo had arrived from the corporate office of the health-care group to which Janice's office belonged. Masks were mandatory in all health-care facilities. They were going to make periodic COVID testing mandatory too.

If a simple mask were a protective tool, then why did everyone declare them useless at the beginning? Janice wondered. Several of her friends were suspicious of wearing them. Everywhere on social media and in public places, anti-masking protesters were calling the mask mandates a violation of their freedom and rights.

A vocal portion of the populace refused to accept the public health statements that masks were effective at thwarting the coronavirus. The anti-mask videos and pictures were widespread on various social media platforms. Janice did not like masks, but she was also afraid for her children.

What if some anti-mask zealot transmitted the virus to her or her kids? What if she got sick? Who would care for her two children if something happened to her? She shuddered at that thought. She was finding it difficult to avoid growing resentment toward people who refused to use masks when, at the very least, wearing a mask couldn't hurt. How selfish can people be? she thought. Even though she didn't like wearing the masks, she had sewn a set of beautiful, soft, and comfortable masks for her children, Leah and Eric.

Later, Janice hurried Leah and Eric into her minivan.

Eric. "Where are we going, Mommy?"

Janice. "We are out of food, hon. I think we need to streamline our grocery shopping to stock up again.

Leah. Are we supposed to wear our masks, Mamma?

Janice. "Yes, sweetie. Remember to sanitize and wear our masks before stepping out in the supermarket.

The supermarket was quite busy, but people stood at a distance in the queue line. Janice and the children shopped quickly, gathering necessities and then hurrying to the cash counter.

She pushed her cart into the parking lot toward the van. A crowd of about a hundred people carrying signs and wearing red hats were shouting slogans. Janice steered her children around the periphery of the crowd. No one was wearing any masks.

Eric. Mommy, why are so many people gathered here without wearing a mask?

Leah. They are not wearing masks, Mamma. All of us will get sick and die soon.

Janice. No, honey. You just keep your mask on and stay close to me.

Janice was mad. They don't have a right to do this. They should respect these rules that are made for their own betterment and safety and to reduce risk to others, she thought.

From a distance, she noticed Agatha, her neighbor from two houses down the street. She was waving a sign that read, "My Body, My Right, My Freedom." Her son, Richard, was there loudly yelling an anti-mask slogan. Janice ushered her children into the van and hurriedly drove away.

Two weeks later, the siren of an ambulance pierced the quiet street of Janice's house. Janice peered out through her window. Agatha and her husband were standing at their door as EMTs rushed into their house. She was sobbing with a mask on her face, and her husband held her close. Minutes later, first responders rolled Richard out in a gurney into the ambulance. An EMT had an Ambu Bag over his face, and he was ventilating the man.

One week later, Richard died due to COVID-19 pneumonia, respiratory failure, and multi-organ system failure. He was thirty-two years old.

Us versus Them

Now in 2023, recommendations by the CDC on masks reflects a more nuanced and comprehensive approach.[19] But back in 2020, the shifting sands of the guidance played out on a desert of poor information about the virus and its transmissibility and infectivity. Between March 2020 and December 2020, the scientific establishment was still grappling with the pathogenic mechanism of the virus as it interacted with its human host. For the first time, science was being faced with the need to perform research and speak with authority about data that was far from proven fact. The obvious hesitancy of public health authorities when it came to making hard factual pronouncements and guidance was counterposed only by the baseless confidence demonstrated by the political leadership in the country.

At the ground level, this constant conflict between the scientific establishment and the anti-fact, anti-science, alternative facts pronouncements of the political establishment created some serious dilemmas on how best to educate and protect the masses of patients who were coming to our clinic doors desperate for the rock of safety and surety.[20] The pandemic, with its universal threat to life and liberty, stripped away the veneer of civilization and unmasked the character of populations. Individuals segregated along fault lines of personalities into broad categories. One group, which I shall call Group A, was characterized by high indices of generalized fear, institutional mistrust, and reliance on self-deterministic approaches to navigating the uncertainty of life. The other, Group B, was characterized by high reliance on collaboration, interdependence, group safety, and acceptance of institutional guidance

---

[19] G. M. Massetti, B. R. Jackson, J. T. Brooks, et al. "Summary of Guidance for Minimizing the Impact of COVID-19 on Individual Persons, Communities, and Health Care Systems—United States," *MMWR Morb Mortal Wkly Rep* 71 (August 2022): 1,057–1,064, http://dx.doi.org/10.15585/mmwr.mm7133e1.

[20] Amy Mitchell, Mark Jurkowitz, J. Baxter Oliphant, and Elisa Shearer. "How Americans Navigated the News in 2020: A Tumultuous Year in Review (Americans inhabited different information environments, with wide gaps in how they viewed the election and COVID-19), Pew Research Center, February 22, 2021.

and control. Unfortunately, both groups would be let down by their champions.

A psychosocial phenomenon called "confirmation bias" ran rampant during this period. Confirmation bias is defined by psychologist Raymond Nickerson as the tendency to search for, interpret, favor, and recall information in a way that confirms or supports one's prior beliefs or values.[21] Confirmation bias was widespread in the way information would be selectively used to support a preferred narrative. A common theme amid the Republican leadership was the narrative of "us versus them." The worldview of this narrative was that America was under siege and under threat of losing its greatness. This was the primary narrative of the Trump administration since 2016, and this narrative appealed to white America's perception of lost or fading greatness.

Having raised the specter of imminent doom, the next theme was the assigning of blame. Thus, "They are responsible for the loss of … for this situation." The second part of this narrative was evident in 2017 by the "Muslim travel ban," by the forcible separation of families at the Southern border, and by the repeal of the DACA policy.[22] In each case, the approach was based on a perception that white America must be preserved and saved from the onslaught of black and brown hordes assailing the American dream and way of life.

The Trump administration did not see its role as the governing of

---

[21] Raymond S. Nickerson, "Confirmation Bias: A Ubiquitous Phenomenon in Many Guises," *Review of General Psychology* 2, no. 2 (1998): 175–220.

[22] Executive Office of the President, "Protecting the Nation from Terrorist Entry into the United States," National Archives, Federal Register, February 1, 2017, https://www.federalregister.gov/documents/2017/02/01/2017-02281/protecting-the-nation-from-foreign-terrorist-entry-into-the-united-states ("Muslim travel ban"); Julie Davis, Julie Hirschfeld, and Michael D. Shear, "How Trump Came to Enforce a Practice of Separating Migrant Families," *The New York Times*, June 16, 2018, archived from the original on June 18, 2018, *retrieved June 19, 2018* (forcible separation of families); and Homeland Security, Office of the Press Secretary, "Recission of Deferred Action for Childhood Arrivals (DACA)," September 5, 2017, https://www.dhs.gov/news/2017/09/05/rescission-deferred-action-childhood-arrivals-daca (DACA repeal).

America to address basic issues of societal growth and equity. Instead, issues such as education, jobs, economy, and opportunity were important only to the extent that these could be preserved and amplified for white America. So, when January 2020 rolled around, and a deadly virus floated across America's borders, the situation was tailor-made for the us-versus-them narrative of the administration. At first, it was nothing more than a bad flu.[23] "No problem! It will go away, folks! Nothing to see here!" Then it became the "China virus."[24]

When it became apparent the pandemic would cause serious economic downturn, instead of confronting it head-on with a clear, focused education and public health campaign, the administration sought to deflect and minimize the fallout in an election year by undermining public health guidelines. Mask mandates were obstructed. Social distancing rules flouted. Business lockdowns were opposed. Instead of educating the public on how they could live safely and conduct their business productively, energy and resources were spent by the Trump administration and the Republican party at every turn from January 2020 through December 2022 to actively undermine, oppose, or thwart measured action that could reduce the impact of the pandemic.[25]

If we at our small primary clinic in northern Virginia could remain open and in contact with hundreds of COVID patients and still carry on our business with safety and productivity, then imagine if the same

---

[23] Brad Brooks. March 13, 2020. "Like the flu? Trump's coronavirus messaging confuses public, pandemic researchers say." https://www.reuters.com/article/us-health-coronavirus-mixed-messages/like-the-flu-trumps-coronavirus-messaging-confuses-public-pandemic-researchers-say-idUSKBN2102GY

[24] Deb Reichmann and Terry Tang. March 18, 2020. Associated Press. "Trump dubs Covid-19 "Chinese virus" despit hate crime risks." https://apnews.com/article/donald-trump-ap-top-news-asia-crime-virus-outbreak-a7c233f0b3bcdb72c06cca6271ba6713

[25] Ryan Zamarripa, associate director of Economic Policy Center for American Progress, "5 Ways the Trump Administration's Policy Failures Compounded the Coronavirus-Induced Economic Crisis," The Center for American Progress, June 3, 2020. https://www.americanprogress.org/article/5-ways-trump-administrations-policy-failures-compounded-coronavirus-induced-economic-crisis/

simple commonsense measures instituted by us had been propagated and implemented by a well-articulated public health campaign and broad education effort that had the enthusiastic support of all the arms of the government without interference and obstruction. One can only imagine how greatly the death toll could have been minimized and how, instead of being a lone beacon of sanctuary on a vast field of us-versus-them devastation, we could have collectively been a vibrant, healthy nation caring and supporting each other through the pandemic.

A Harvest of Fear

The United States has only 4 percent of the world's population and yet experienced 15 percent of the global COVID-19 mortality. To the immediate north, Canada, which had a unified public health initiative and a unified governmental response, had a per capita COVID-19 death rate through February 2021 of two hundred thousand fewer deaths than the United States.[26] This single statistic alone is the most damning indictment of US Republican leadership from 2016 to 2020, and history is likely to judge their performance as a criminal dereliction of duty.

The sad irony of this is that the same anti-vax, anti-science, conspiracy theorist-proposing narratives that damaged the US public health response resulted in more Republicans dying of COVID before vaccines were available due to their resistance to public health mitigation efforts.[27] Later, when the first vaccines rolled out, far fewer Republicans opted to receive COVID vaccination. As a result, Republicans died in greater numbers than did Democrats.[28] A study conducted by Paul

---

[26] T. Campbell, A. P. Galvani, G. Friedman, and M. C. Fitzpatrick, "Exacerbation of COVID-19 Mortality by the Fragmented United States Healthcare System: A Retrospective Observational Study," *Lancet Reg Health Am* 12 (August 2022): 100,264.

[27] Annabelle Timsit, "Washington State Senator Doug Ericksen Dies after Battling COVID-19," *Washington Post*, December 19, 2021.

[28] Jacob Wallace, Paul Goldsmith-Pinkham, and Jason L. Schwartz, "Excess Death Rates for Republicans and Democrats during the COVID-19 Pandemic,"

Goldsmith-Pinkham, Jacob Wallace, and Jason L. Schwartz of the Yale School of Public Health found that Republicans paid a higher price in COVID mortality both before and after vaccines became available, but the divergence in excess mortality rates in the post-vaccination period between Republicans and Democrats was even more striking.[29] Indeed, in the history that will be written of these pandemic years, it cannot fail to be noted that the grim reaper did harvest more of the heads of those who embraced the policies of fear, division, and disruption than of those who turned, instead, to fact and fellowship. This essential feature of the pandemic years is inescapable to almost everyone involved with caring for the sick populace in the trenches. The section that follows contains a post I wrote in a newsletter to my patients; it was an exhortation to keep the faith in humanity and human goodness during particularly bleak moments.

The Power of Faith

The greatest casualty of 2020 was the loss of faith in the beneficence of public institutions. The value of faith as an instrument of well-being was not always clear to me when I began my career. As a physician, I was trained in the scientific method. I was taught to use the powers of my intellect in the service of the human condition. Later, during my postdoctoral years at Harvard, this exaltation of the capacity of

---

National Bureau of Economic Research, Working Paper Series, No. 30512, September 2022, https://www.nber.org/papers/w30512; Robert Zullo, "Virginia State Senator Dies of COVID-19 Complications," *Virginia Mercury*, January 1, 2021; Claudia Grisales, "Rep. Ron Wright is 1st Member of Congress to Die after Coronavirus Diagnosis," *NPR*, February 8, 2021; Gabriel San Roman, "Kelly Ernby, Former Orange County GOP State Assembly Candidate and Deputy DA Dies of COVID-19," *Los Angeles Times*, January 3, 2022; and Brian Bakst and Kirsti Marohn, "Minn. Sen. Jerry Relph Dies of COVID-19 complications," *MPRNews*, December 18, 2020.

[29] Wallace, Goldsmith-Pinkham, and Schwartz, "Excess Death Rates for Republicans and Democrats."

dispassionate observation and worship at the altar of measurable metrics was honed to even higher degrees. Thus, even though I wrote each prescription prefaced with the ancient script "Rx" as the symbolic last remnant of the ancient physician's prayer, "Take thou in the name of God," the question of faith never entered into the operations of diagnosis and treatment of disease.

But then life has a wonderful way of doubling you back on yourself and making you come face-to-face with your greatest denials. I did not have to be a doctor for too long during this pandemic before I was confronted with the essential question of faith. What is it? I wondered. And do we really need it to live productively? Indeed, without proceeding so far as to ever invoke the existence of a higher power, this much has become very clear to me as I have worked with the sick, dying, and panic-stricken during this pandemic.

We human beings exist every minute based on faith. It is faith that allows us to release our grip on each exhaled breath with no guarantee we will be able to inhale the next lungful. It is faith that protects a child from fear when he waves goodbye to his dad or mom with the confidence he will see them again that evening. It is faith that forms the foundation of the constancy of affection between a man and a woman. Every step we take, every gesture we make, every sound we speak is made based on a faith that reality will continue to proceed along predictable probabilities.

Yet we live in a society that continues to scoff at faith even as those who scoff use faith to ground themselves. I sometimes wonder at the colossal magnitude of this self-deception. But I find I seldom have too much time to stand and wonder at such folk. My waiting room is full each day with tired and fevered souls who come to my door with the faith that I would better their woe. And most times, I find that, despite intellectual knowledge of my limitations, their faith inspires me to accomplish what they hope. Indeed, to serve as a physician is to practice the artful application of faith for the weal of humanity.

Thus, it is in this simple fact that I see the true power of faith revealed. For truly the phenomenon of faith is the lasting sign that we are not beings of clay destined to dissolve in dust but, rather, glorious blazes of hope, light, and energy that fashion our world with the power of our committed belief. Faith is not some blind illusion but, instead, a glorious vision of our daily triumph over the bonds of cloying matter. Faith in the form of the steadfast intention of a father is what makes a son manifest that intent. Faith in the form of the resolute night vigil of a mother is what makes a fevered child open its eyes to see the morn. The words "I believe" are the substance of redemption from blind repetition of the past. Hope is not a dull opiate of denial from confronting reality. A life without faith is impossible to live no matter how loudly you may protest that you do not believe. The halls of mental institutions are filled with the shells of terrified souls who have lost faith. A life lived in denial of faith is equal to one who willfully chooses to poison the very well that sustains him. And it is in recognition of this truth that all rituals and celebrations practiced by all religions have their basis.

That faith is not to be found in a temple, a synagogue, a mosque or a church, but in each breath, we take, each dream we cherish, each plan we make, each glance we cast, each hand we hold, and each tear we wipe.

CHAPTER 4

The Face of the Reaper

*If you know the enemy and know yourself, you need not
fear the result of a hundred battles. If you know yourself
but not the enemy, for every victory gained you will also
suffer a defeat. If you know neither the enemy nor yourself,
you will succumb in every battle.*

—Sun Tzu, Art of War

An Ancient Evil

Coronaviruses are ancient, with one paper dating them back millions of
years old.[30] All viruses are essentially snippets of genetic material packaged
within a protein coat.[31] The genetic material or nucleic acid strand in a
virus may be DNA (deoxyribonucleic acid) or RNA (ribonucleic acid).
Coronaviruses are RNA viruses, and their genetic material contains the
instructions the virus uses to commandeer the infected cells' biochemical
machinery to create more copies of itself. The copies of the viral nucleic

---

[30] J. O. Wertheim, D. K. Chu, J. S. Peiris, S. L. Kosakovsky Pond, and L. L. Poon,
"A Case for the Ancient Origin of Coronaviruses," *J Virol* 87, no. 12 (June 2013):
7,039–45, doi: 10.1128/JVI.03273-12, epub April 17, 2013, PMID: 23596293,
PMCID: PMC3676139.
[31] Jane Flint, Vincent R. Racaniello, Glenn F. Rall, Theodora Hatziioannou, and
Anna Marie Skalka, *Principles of Virology*, multivolume 5th ed. (Wiley & Sons).

acid are packaged by the infected cell into protein envelopes of new viral particles, and the virions burst out of the hapless infected cell to infect additional host cells and begin a new cycle of infection, replication, and propagation.

A virus is essentially a pure genetic code. Viruses do not contain any of the complex metabolic machinery we see in all higher cells and organisms. Instead, a virus uses the host cells' machinery to execute its code. The ability of a viral particle to infect a host cell is determined by small protein molecules on the surface of the viral particle that recognize and lock onto specific protein receptor molecules on the host cell. This property is called tropism ("affinity"), and viruses have evolved over millions of years to display exquisite tropism for specific cells based on the mutual specificity of recognition and affinity between the viral envelope protein and the host surface receptor. The host surface receptor is usually a host cellular protein that serves some vital function for the host and the virus has evolved a surface recognition protein that happens to recognize and attach to the host receptor. Consider the situation as a specific housebreaking tool created by a burglar to jimmy or crack open a specific door or window latch to enter a house.

The "house latch" that the SARS-CoV-2 virus has developed as a tool to housebreak is the ACE2 (angiotensin- converting enzyme 2) receptor, a vital surface protein widely present in all mammalian cells across species. The ACE2 receptor serves such a vital function that its structure is "evolutionarily conserved" across all mammalian species; this means the ACE2 receptor of a bat is very similar in structure to that of a human. Evolutionary conservation is seen in all molecules that serve such important functions to a cell that modification of their structure would usually be catastrophic to the cell. From a burglar's perspective, evolutionarily conserved host molecules means that a housebreaking tool developed against a conserved host molecule of one species will likely work to housebreak into a cell of another species. This cross-species utility is the basis of an animal virus's ability to jump species from one animal to another and from an animal to a human. When this happens, it is said that the virus has "gained a function" and forms the basis of understanding the controversy over NIH-funded "gain-of-function" scientific research that was the subject of much heated debate and congressional hearings during the pandemic.[32]

A Crown of Thorns

Coronaviruses are a vast family with a wide distribution in the animal kingdom. There are different coronaviruses specific to bats, lions, tigers, giraffes, camels, civets, and even dolphins and beluga whales.

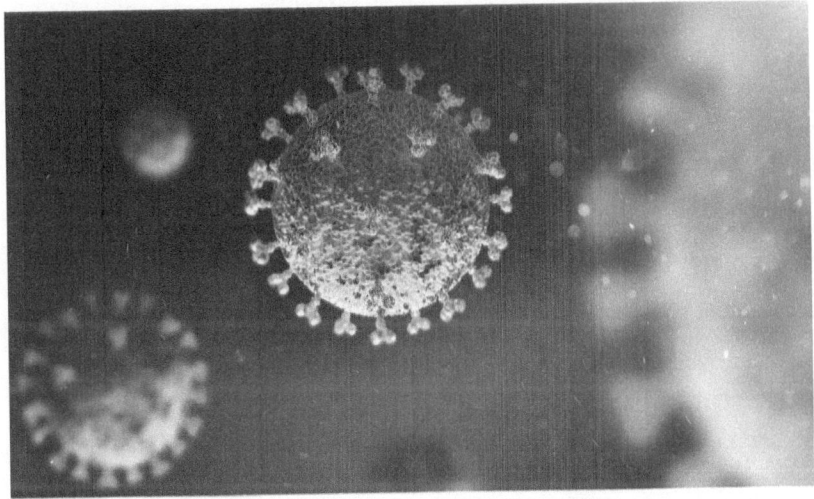

There are seven coronaviruses that infect humans, and these belong to the alpha and beta coronavirus families that also infect bats, pigs, cats, dogs, horses, mice, rats, rabbits, cows, antelope, giraffe, camels, civets, and badgers. The "corona" of these viruses comes from the spiky "crown of thorns" appearance of the surface of these viruses under an electron microscope, and these spike proteins are the determinants of the

---

[32] Senate Homeland Security and Governmental Affairs, Hearings to Examine Gain of Function Research, Focusing on What the Pandemic Taught Us and Where to Go from Here, August 3, 2022, 117th Congress (2021–2022), https://www.congress.gov/event/117th-congress/senate-event/332968?s=1&r=8.

attachment to the host mammalian cell. Both the original SARS-CoV virus of the SARS epidemic of 2003 and the SARS-CoV-2 virus of the COVID-19 pandemic attach to the ACE2 receptor on the surface of human and bat cells and belong to the beta coronavirus family. Unlike the SARS-CoV-2 virus that causes COVID-19, there is no vaccine or treatment currently available for the 2003 SARS virus.

Our understanding of the SARS-CoV-2 virus has evolved exponentially in the past two and half years.[33] Within sixty days of formal recognition (at the end of November 2019) of the novel coronavirus SARS-CoV-2 and the disease COVID-19 that it caused, scientists had the full sequenced genome available. SARS-CoV-2 is closely related to 2003 SARS-CoV.[34] It is 96 percent identical at the whole genomic level to the bat coronavirus strain BatCoV Ra TG13. The homology at the structural protein level is even higher, with the structural M glycoprotein of the virus being 98 percent homologous between bat, pangolin, and human strains of the virus.[35]

It is this homology that is the basis of the postulate that the original BatCoV Ra TG13 virus may have jumped species by way of pangolins to humans and that the place this may have occurred is the Wuhan wet market, where live animals of both of the first two species were sold and consumed by the third. Bats are ecologically separated from humans, so such a crossover requires exposure and contact. The phenomenon of

---

[33] American Society for Microbiology, "SARS-CoV-2 Sequencing Data: The Devil Is in the Genomic Detail," ASM website, October 28, 2020, https://asm.org/Articles/2020/October/SARS-CoV-2-Sequencing-Data-The-Devil-Is-in-the-Gen#:~:text=In%20January%202020%2C%20when%20an,scientists%20immediately%20sequenced%20its%20genome.

[34] N. Zhu, D. Zhang, W. Wang, X. Li, B. Yang, J. Song, X. Zhao, B. Huang, W. Shi, R. Lu, P. Niu, F. Zhan, X. Ma, D. Wang, W. Xu, G. Wu, G. F. Gao, and W, Tan, "China Novel Coronavirus Investigating and Research Team: A Novel Coronavirus from Patients with Pneumonia in China, 2019," *N Engl J Med* 382, no. 8 (February 20, 2020): 727–33.

[35] S. Thomas, "The Structure of the Membrane Protein of SARS-CoV-2 Resembles the Sugar Transporter SemiSWEET," *Pathog Immun* 5, no. 1 (October 19, 2020): 342–63.

zoonotic viral outbreaks is a well-known phenomenon in countries where bush meat is consumed.[36] The key in a zoonotic viral outbreak is the opportunity for transfer of the virus from its natural animal reservoir in which the virus is endemic to another species that is not the virus's normal host. When such transfer occurs, the probability of the virus acquiring new functions as it adapts to its new host is very high, and such an event may result in an eventual gain of function capability to infect humans.

The two prior coronavirus outbreaks had taken precisely such a path. The 2003 SARS-CoV outbreak had emerged from bats and jumped to humans by way of an intermediary host of palm civet cats.[37] The 2012 MERS (Middle East respiratory syndrome) virus similarly emerged from bats and jumped to humans by way of dromedary camels.[38] The host receptor that is targeted for viral attachment and entry in SARS-CoV and SARS-CoV-2 is the ACE2 receptor, while for the MERS virus it is the DPP4 receptor.

Indeed, as forest decline and ecological degradation due to deforestation, human development, and climate change continue, the opportunity for zoonotic microbial and viral outbreaks exponentially escalates, as humans in impoverished regions of the world come in increasing contact with wild animal populations. In addition, as climate change devastates agricultural yields, nutritional pressure will drive human populations toward increasing consumption of alternate

---

[36] L. A. Kurpiers, B. Schulte-Herbrüggen, I. Ejotre, and D. M. Reeder, "Bushmeat and Emerging Infectious Diseases: Lessons from Africa," *Problematic Wildlife*, (September 21, 2015): 507–551.

[37] S. K. Lau, "Ecoepidemiology and Complete Genome Comparison of Different Strains of Severe Acute Respiratory Syndrome-Related Rhinolophus Bat Coronavirus in China Reveal Bats as a Reservoir for Acute, Self-Limiting Infection That Allows Recombination Events," *J. Virol.* 84 no. 6 (2010): 2,808–2819 and W. Li W, "Bats Are Natural Reservoirs of SARS-like Coronaviruses," *Science* 310, no. 5,748 (2005): 676–79.

[38] A. Zumla, D. S. Hui, and S. Perlman, "Middle East Respiratory Syndrome," *Lancet* 386, no. 9,997 (September 5, 2015): 995–1,007.

nutritional sources such as bush meat and game consumption, making zoonotic outbreaks virtually inevitable in our futures.

The Spike

The attachment of the SARS-CoV-2 virus to the cells of the respiratory epithelium occurs by a specific interaction between the viral spike protein and the ACE2 receptor on the human cell.[39] The viral spike protein consists of an S1 unit that is furthest away from the viral surface and an S2 unit that forms a stalk connected to the viral surface. The three copies of the S1-S2 monomer are assembled into a trimer that constitutes the final spike protein.

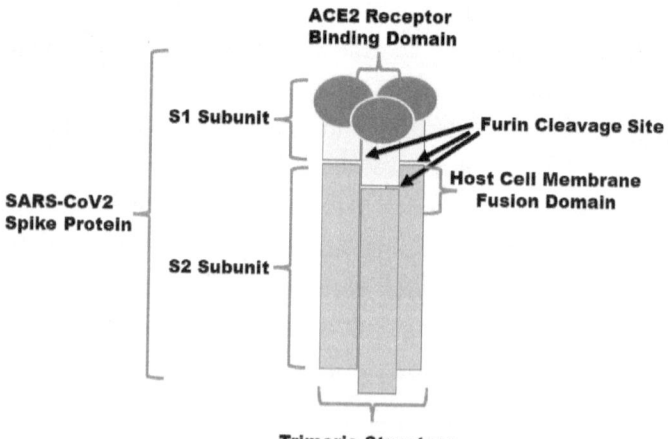

Figure 4.1: SARS-CoV2 Spike Protein Schematic Structure

---

[39] Cong Xu, Yanxing Wang, Caixuan Liu, Chao Zhang, Wenyu Han, Xiaoyu Hong, Yifan Wang, Qin Hong, Shutian Wang, Qiaoyu Zhao, Yalei Wang, Yong Yang, Kaijian Chen, Wei Zheng, Liangliang Kong, Fangfang Wang, Qinyu Zuo, Zhong Huang, and Yao Cong, "Conformational Dynamics of SARS-CoV-2 Trimeric Spike Glycoprotein in Complex with Receptor ACE2 Revealed by cryo-EM," *Science Advances* 7, no. 1 (January 1, 2021) and J. Lan, J. Ge, J. Yu, *et al.*, "Structure of the SARS-CoV-2 Spike Receptor-Binding Domain Bound to the ACE2 Receptor," *Nature* 581 (2020): 215–20 (2020), https://doi.org/10.1038/s41586-020-2180-5.

The S1 unit contains the receptor binding domain (RBD) that determines the attachment to the ACE2 receptor, while the S2 unit is responsible for fusion of the virus with the human cell and the entry of the virus into the human cell. Fusion with and entry of the virus into the human cell requires the S1 unit of the spike protein to be separated from the S2 unit and, this separation is mediated by a human serine-protease enzyme closely associated with the ACE2 receptor. The point of cleavage between the S1 and S2 units is called the furin cleavage site. So, essentially, the process of viral infection of the human cell is a two-part process, the first being a binding of the S1 unit to the human ACE2 receptor.[40] This is followed by cleavage of the S1 from the S2 unit at the furin cleavage site, which activates the S2 unit to begin fusion of the viral particle with the human cell and entry of the virus into the human cell.

Mutations that alter the structure of spike protein subunits produce variants that differ in their virulence and in their ability to evade neutralization by antibodies. For example, the enhanced transmissibility of the delta variant that emerged in India in December 2020 had mutations in the spike protein that resulted in making the furin cleavage site more accessible to cleavage, allowing for easier S2 unit activation with resultant enhanced transmissibility of the delta variant.[41]

The interaction of a virus with the human system is a fascinating story of life's perpetual struggle for dominance and survival. Every viral particle comes under attack by the human system, and every virus has evolved various strategies for escape from this attack. There are seven escape strategies known in the SARS-CoV-2 virus:[42]

1. Camouflage of the spike proteins by sugar molecules to evade recognition.

[40] Fang Tian, Bei Tong, Liang Sun, Shengchao Shi, Bin Zheng, Zibin Wang, Xianchi Dong, and Peng Zheng, "N501Y Mutation of Spike Protein in SARS-CoV-2 Strengthens Its Binding to Receptor ACE2," *eLife* 10 (2021): e69091, https://doi.org/10.7554/eLife.69091.

[41] A. Rubio-Casillas, E. M. Redwan, and V. N. Uversky, "SARS-CoV-2: A Master of Immune Evasion," *Biomedicines* 10, no. 6 (June 7, 2022): 1,339.

[42] Fang Tian et al., "N501Y Mutation of Spike Protein in SARS-CoV-2."

2. Direct interference of the mechanisms by which portions of viral proteins are cut up by the human system and presented to the immune system by a sophisticated molecular immune recognition system called MHC-I antigen presentation.

3. Inhibition of synthesis of a human immune cytokine called interferon that teaches immune cells to attack the virus.

4. Viral interference of a human cellular defense mechanism called "apoptysis" that would result in viral-infected cells committing accelerated death, a kind of cellular suicide, rather than serve as viral replication factories.

5. Direct cell-to-cell infection promoted by viral-infected human cells to directly connect with neighboring cells through cellular nanotubes to directly transmit infective virus to adjacent cells through these channels and, thereby, evade exposure to the immune system cells lurking outside.

6. Direct cell-to-cell infection by web formation of connections (syncytia formation) between virus-infected and uninfected cells.

7. Release of infective virus from infected human cells in cellular blebs called exosomes that fuse with neighboring uninfected cells, thereby bypassing the ACE2 receptor-mediated attachment and entry mechanism and allowing for infection into human cells and tissue that may not express the ACE2 receptor on their surface.

A FaceTime Farewell

Early in the pandemic, scientists understood the virus was inhaled into the respiratory tract by aerosolized droplets of sneeze or cough secretions from infected individuals. It was also well understood that people were disseminating high loads of virus for three to five days before they themselves developed symptoms significant enough to alert them to the presence of the disease.

The virus was attaching to the ACE2 receptor molecules on human cells lining the respiratory tract by way of the receptor-binding domain of the S1 subunit of the viral spike protein. A human cell surface enzyme present in association with the ACE2 receptor then cleaved the viral spike protein at the furin cleavage point between the S1 and S2 subunits of the viral spike protein. Cleavage allowed the S1 unit to separate from the S2 unit, and the exposed S2 unit was now activated to begin the process of fusing the virus with the human cell. This ended in entry of the virus into the human cell and passage of the viral genetic material into the human cell, where it would be read by the human gene-reading machinery, and the instructions contained in the viral genome would be faithfully carried out.

The viral genetic material was replicated, and new virions were packaged, which then burst forth to infect the adjacent cells. The process was one of exponential progressions, like a wildfire through the lungs. Infected cells swelled and exploded, releasing an explosion of virions like so many pieces of shrapnel to pierce adjacent cells. Viremia developed as billions of viral particles entered the bloodstream and penetrated every organ, nook, and cranny of the body.

The damaged and dying cells released chemical signals that brought in a flood of the body's defenses. These defensive cells of the body, neutrophils, macrophages and monocytes, B lymphocytes, and T lymphocytes flooded into the lung in response to the chemical signals released by bursting respiratory tissue cells. A battle royale was being waged in a take-no-prisoner war in the lungs of the hapless victims. Fluids and secretions began to build up in the lung—the cellular equivalent of a river of blood flowing on a battlefield of dead and dying infected respiratory cells. The air grew dank and fetid as the fresh breeze of life was choked and clogged in swollen, congested airways. Oxygen, the essence of life, was no longer able to flow past mounting heaps of cellular debris swollen with secretions. Blood oxygenation levels began to drop as O2 saturations plummeted to 70 to 80 percent, levels far below when people would qualify for being put on a ventilator.

Meanwhile, the body's defense armies were on a rampage. Driven wild by a barrage of triggers from an avalanche of viral proteins being released from infected cells, the human immune system went nuclear, unleashing a massive surge of some of its most potent chemical arsenal in what has been termed "the cytokine storm." The scorched-earth campaign of a molecular apocalypse had begun. The interleukin cytokines IL-1, IL-2, IL-6 and a dozen others, along with TNF-alfa (tumor necrosis factor-alfa), spread indiscriminately through the body unleashing havoc. Tissues and cells in uninfected organs began to swell and die under the toxic fire of this chemical holocaust.

The clotting system was activated without any restraint, and the blood all over the body began to congeal in the tiny capillaries of distant organs and tissues. The dreaded march of DIC (disseminated intravascular coagulation) had begun. It was as if a thousand microscopic heart attacks were happening all over the body. In the lung, heart, kidney, skin, gut, brain, liver, muscle, and bone, clots plugged blood vessels, denying vital blood flow to healthy tissue. The body, unable to eradicate the virus, was performing the ultimate sacrifice to protect not itself but, rather, the fate of humanity. It was imploding in an act of organismal suicide of the infected, disease-ridden body so the still healthy specimens of humanity may have a fighting chance at survival.

And so, trapped in an ICU with their faces encased in an elephantine trunk of ventilator flex tubing, millions of hapless victims gasped their last breaths, attended by a nurse dressed in an astronaut moon suit, while their family said their wailing declarations of love and goodbyes through the cellular screens of an iPhone FaceTime farewell.

ICU Day 15

The nurse steps in to check on the woman in the bed. She is barely visible, lying there somewhere beneath the tangled maze of ventilator and intravenous tubing. Above her, a fluorescent green blip dances its way across the screen of a monitor. Yellow numbers glow out readings of pulse, blood pressure, and oxygen saturation level. The room is filled with the low hiss of the ventilator motor.

On the window ledge, an iPhone plays a soft playlist through a small

Bluetooth speaker. But the woman in ICU bed number 5 does not notice it. She is sedated, deep under a propofol-induced sleep, blissfully unconscious of the disease that is ravaging her body—that has ravaged her body.

Now, only the chemical cocktail of the drugs dripping in her veins and the mechanical beat of the ventilator are forcing her life force into being a reluctant tenant in a body fast approaching the point of becoming a dwelling incompatible with life.

I have been this woman's doctor for many years. She did everything right. She isolated, washed hands, covered her face, and stayed away from crowds. Her husband, daughter, and son all followed my guidance to a T. Pity that the rest of her friends did not. Too bad the neighbors on her street did not. Somewhere out there, someone had felt they had a greater right to their breath of maskless fresh air. So, this forty-eight-year-old, beautiful wife and mother will have to give up her right to all her breaths. A fifty-year-old man will have to watch the love of his life struggle to give up her ghost through a cell phone video, and a teenage son and a daughter will spend the rest of their lives without the breath of a mother fanning their cheeks.

The Naked Emperor

All this knowledge about the general viral mechanisms of infection and attack was present in the global scientific community even before the onset of the pandemic, and the specific mechanisms used by SARS-CoV-2 was well understood by March 2020. But none of this knowledge was used to craft a simple, effective public health policy and public education campaign in the United States because the leadership in the United States possessed the intellectual capacity for comprehension of an elementary school child. When you have the president of the United States opining on the value of irradiating UV light inside lungs and of injecting bleach and disinfectant into lungs and body tissue as if human beings were so many objects of furniture to be wiped free and disinfected, then you can begin to comprehend the colossal knowledge deficit the country was operating under.[43]

My patients in my clinic had access to much greater comprehensive guidance and knowledge about viral mechanisms and methods of prevention and safety than the White House coronavirus briefings in 2020. What was tragic was that no one had the courage to call this out. The emperor was prancing down Pennsylvania Avenue in naked, narcissistic splendor attended by fawning self-serving courtiers, and no one could turn their stunned gaze from the horrific spectacle long enough to declare the obvious before them all.

Everyone kept trying to "manage" the buffoon in the house, in the hope that, somehow, the damage could be mitigated and contained. From papers that would be whisked away to briefings that would be tailored, long before the pandemic, US policy was being crafted by a shadow government of public servant managers who had decided they had to quietly save America from the Nero at its helm.[44] Before and after the pandemic started, the media focused on what was most important to the media — "ratings"! Whether it was the liberal media or the conservative media, the focus was always the ratings value of the circus show of Pennsylvania Avenue, with policy and facts playing second fiddle.

All over the world morgues were overflowing. Graveyards were running out of space. The dead were being buried lying on their sides so graves could be cut narrower, and more bodies stacked per square yard of terrain. In India and other parts of Southeast Asia, crematoriums were melting down in the relentless heat of nonstop cremations, and firewood

---

[43] Dartunoro Clark. April 23, 2020. NBC News. "Trump suggests 'injection' of disinfectant to beat coronavirus and 'clean' the lung." https://www.nbcnews.com/politics/donald-trump/trump-suggests-injection-disinfectant-beat-coronavirus-clean-lungs-n1191216.

[44] Philip Rucker and Robert Costa, "Bob Woodward's New Book Reveals a 'Nervous Breakdown' of Trump's Presidency," *Washington Post*, September 4, 2018, https://www.washingtonpost.com/politics/bob-woodwards-new-book-reveals-a-nervous-breakdown-of-trumps-presidency/2018/09/04/b27a389e-ac60-11e8-a8d7-0f63ab8b1370_story.html.

was running out for crematoriums. Globally, a hundred Romes were burning. The fires of hell were blazing, and the devil and his minions were dancing in an inferno fueled by a growing field of corpses scythed down by a reaper wearing a crown of spikes.

CHAPTER 5

Pandora's Tears

When Pandora saw inside the box, she cried black acid for tears.
        —Lara Croft: Tomb Raider—The Cradle of Life

The Final Gasp

Rachel had been working nonstop for eighteen hours in this ER. Three other nurses were down with COVID, one was upstairs in the ICU on a vent, and so Rachel was pulling two straight shifts and going into her third. The waiting room was overflowing with sick people who needed quick treatment. The hospital was in chaos. Patients were lined up in the hallway, their breathing labored and strained. Nurses and doctors rushed from bed to bed, trying their best to keep up with the influx of patients. But it was like holding back an ocean. There simply weren't enough resources to go around, and patients were dying every day.

The entire city of New York had been severely affected by the COVID-19 pandemic, and the hospital was overrun. An exhausted ER physician walked up to Rachel. His face looked drawn and tired. His shirt was open at the neck, and he didn't bother to hide the two-day, unshaven stubble that darkened his jawline.

In one corner of the room, a young man lay on a hospital bed, alone, an oxygen face mask hissing on his face. He had been admitted just a few

56

hours before, and his condition was rapidly deteriorating. Rachel bent over another bed. She held up her iPhone to the face of a dying man—a man who was struggling to breathe. His eyes appeared glazed. His skin was gray, and the voices of his family came through the phone's speaker, echoing over the hiss of the respirators. They were crying and praying for a miracle. "We love you, Dad," wailed a weeping voice.

Rachel finished the call and walked out of the room. The hallway was lined with gurneys of gasping patients. She quickly opened a door and stepped into the small room. It was a janitor supply closet. Her chest was heavy, and her head felt faint. Fumbling, she pulled out her phone and called her father in Michigan. He is seventy, she thought, and alone.

Panic rose in her, grabbing her by the throat until, at last, her father's face came on the phone screen. Choking with relief, Rachel spoke to him. Her voice was urgent, concerned. "Don't go out! Wear your mask. Have everything delivered. Don't worry about cost, Dad."

The old man reassured her.

She broke down. Sobbing, she said, "I love you, Daddy." Then she slumped down the wall of the tiny room, sobbing her heart out in the darkness of the closet.

Human beings are a connected species. To be able to connect and to be able to remain connected is our life blood. We rely on establishing this connection through proximity and through touch. Very few of us have developed any meaningful skill at fostering connection through intention or through mental focus. The pandemic, in a single moment, put an end to this connection at a global level and eight billion humans writhed and gasped and languished like so many worms dying under a blazing noonday sun.[45]

---

[45] D. Azim, S. Kumar, S. Nasim, T. B. Arif, and D. Nanjiani, "COVID-19 as a Psychological Contagion: A New Pandora's Box to Close?" *Infect Control Hosp Epidemiol* 41, no. 8 (August 2020): 989–90.

Sleeping with the Enemy

Lena sat outside in her small apartment, tears streaming down her cheeks. She felt alone, abandoned. Her husband, Mike, had just left after another violent outburst. She looked around at the destruction he had caused, the broken vase and overturned furniture a cruel reminder of the reality she lived in. Lena had always felt trapped in her marriage to Mike. He was controlling and abusive, both physically and mentally. But ever since the pandemic and all the lockdowns, things had gotten worse.

Every day felt like a never-ending nightmare for Lena. She was stuck in her small apartment, with no escape from Mike's wrath. He was constantly on edge, his temper flaring at the smallest of things, and Lena was always the target of his animosity.

She whispered to herself in despair, "I can't do this anymore. I can't keep living like this. But where would I go? I have no one who can help me out in this situation."

She was pregnant, and she had not told him yet about it. She was scared to tell him and scared to not tell. Already, she kept her hands close across her torso when Mike had his bursts of rage, unconsciously protecting the unborn life within. All across the world, death was marching the streets, but Lena had to protect just one life. Nothing else.

That evening, she watched Mike, who was searching for something in the walk-in closet. He seemed to be a little distracted.

Lena. What are you looking for?

Mike, exhaling slowly and turning away from Lena. I don't have time to answer your stupid questions.

Lena. Maybe I can help you?

Mike came closer, grabbed her neck, and said, "I'll break your neck if you ever try to speak when I'm busy with something. Stay out of my life." He gave her a sharp look and left the room.

Lena sat down on the edge of the bed and started crying. She had this horrible feeling that something terrible was about to happen. She tried to scream, but no sound would come out.

Bruises Everywhere

I walked into the exam room. Lena was sitting on the table cradling her arm.

"Good morning, Mrs. Rodriguez. Are you OK?" I asked.

"Oh hey, Dr. Iyer. I'm fine. Just had a little accident. I stumbled down the stairs."

But when I examined her, there were bruises everywhere. And slowly at first and then faster in a rush, Lena poured her story out to my nurse and me in our clinic. She talked about the bouts of anger that had started six months after she was married and then worsened once the lockdown started, and Mike had lost his job when the restaurant he worked in closed. She told us how, before, she could go out to work and have at least ten hours of abuse-free existence; now she was locked in the same apartment with her abuser.

Mike would start drinking at noon, and by 3:00 p.m., the beatings would begin. Sometimes, he would simply climb on her and beat her in a sexual rage. Mike didn't need a reason. Lately, he accused Lena of cheating on him.

Sobbing, Lena shared that she was hurt and frustrated. "Dr. Iyer," she said, "I loved Mike, and we had a happy family. But everything changed between us when the pandemic hit. And now our relationship has become a nightmare. I didn't cheat on him, I promise, Dr. Iyer. I could never do that. Please, please, help me. I can't take it anymore."

The story of Lena and Mike was one of the hundreds of thousands of domestic abuse and violence stories that occurred during the pandemic across the world. Locked into a forced existence with their abusers, countless women and children across the world suffered and died. Many survived with deep scars and broken bodies.

It was not only spousal abuse. For reasons still not very clear, COVID affects adults more than it does children. Maybe there exists a differential level of expression of the ACE2 receptor in children compared to adults. Maybe the immune response of children does not devolve into the deadly cytokine storm as frequently as in adults. Whatever the reason, adults were affected, suffered, and died at much higher rates than children. As a result, the number of children who became orphaned by the loss of one or both parents during the pandemic soared globally. Families disintegrated, and humans descended into poverty across the globe as income-generating adults perished by the millions. The effect was especially pronounced on families already just eking out an existence before the pandemic. As poverty rose, so also did predation. Bereft of adult parental protection, minors were engulfed by human trafficking networks. Human trafficking soared during the pandemic.[46]

The apocalyptic four horsemen of food insecurity, financial insecurity, mental insecurity, and physical insecurity rode rampant through global communities in the wake of the fifth horseman of disease.[47] Disease was not the only predatory demon preying on the most vulnerable of humanity.

Lena was successful in escaping her sad circumstances. Together with county resources and police assistance, she was able to break free. Today, she has a job and is raising her one-year-old son. But her story is an illustration that a strong public health policy is not merely about public health. It is about preserving the health metrics of all aspects of a society's existence, from business and economy to human rights and well-being. This is something politicians who profess to lead a nation should never forget.

---

[46] L. Khuluq, S. Sriharini, A. Izudin, and I. Abdullah, "The Manipulation of Power and the Trafficking of Women during the COVID-19 Pandemic: Narratives from Indonesia." *Journal of Human Trafficking* (2022): 1–14; J. Todres and A. Diaz, "COVID-19 and Human Trafficking: The Amplified Impact on Vulnerable Populations," *JAMA Pediatrics* 175, no. 2 (2021), 123–24.

[47] Laura Cordiso Tsai, Joanna Eleccion and Ankita Panda. Journal of Modern Slavery. Vol. 6, Issue 2, 2021. COVID-19 and Modern Slavery. https://slavefreetoday. org/journal_of_modern_slavery/v6i2a11_ImpactoftheCOVID19pandemic onsurvivorsofhumantraffickinginthePhilippines.pdf.

CHAPTER 6

Gain of Function

From inability to let well alone, from too much zeal for the new and contempt for what is old, from putting knowledge before wisdom, science before art and cleverness before common sense, from treating patients as cases and from making the cure of the disease more grievous than the endurance of the same, good Lord deliver us.
—Sir Robert Hutchison, "The Physician's Prayer"

Early Warnings

The process by which a virus natural to an animal host acquires the ability to infect a human requires the virus to acquire new capabilities to bind with human cell surface receptors and use human cellular machinery for its replication and propagation or, in essence, a "gain of function." This process can occur randomly in nature by just chance exposure, though in actuality, this leap from the natural animal reservoir of a virus to a human host often requires an intermediary host animal to facilitate the acquisition of these new human-specific functions. The process of such events is, fortunately, far from common. But ecological degradation and climate change has been altering the equation toward increasing the probability of such an event. Still, there have been prescient minds in the scientific community ringing the alarm bells of the risk of viral pandemics for years.

Experts and public figures have been variously warning of pandemic unpreparedness, pandemic vulnerabilities and risks and pandemic inevitability since 2005.[48, 49, 50, 51] Indeed the growing ability of scientists to manipulate the genome of organisms by inserting foreign genes or deleting endogenous genes or splicing genes from other species to create chimeric organisms with novel biologic properties has raised alarm in both scientists, regulatory agencies and knowledgeable members of the public. Developments as early as 2001 by Jackson et al. who developed a strain of mousepox that overcame both natural disease induced and vaccine immunity along with the separate complete synthesis of the polio virus made it clear that humankind had the potential to unleash upon itself a catastrophe of unimaginable proportions.

These fears were given impetus in 2011, when scientists Yoshihiro Kawaoka, and Ron Fouchier, independently demonstrated a cross species jump of the avian influenza virus from birds to mammalian ferrets by repeatedly infecting ferrets with the avian virus. Such repeated exposure allowed the viruses to acquire the capability to spontaneously spread as a respiratory virus between ferrets without the aid of manual infection by the scientists. In addition, the mutations that the viruses had acquired in the process of adaptation to the cooler respiratory passages of the ferrets also conferred upon them the ability to be transmitted from one

[48] M. T. Osterholm, "[Preparing for the Next Pandemic]," *Salud Publica de Mexico 48, no. 3 (*2005): 279–85.

[49] H. Chen, G. J. D. Smith, K. S. Li, J. Wang, X. H. Fan, J. M. Rayner, D. Vijaykrishna, J. X. Zhang, L. J. Zhang, C. T. Guo, C. L. Cheung, K. M. Xu, L. Duan, K. Huang, K. Qin, Y. H. C. Leung, W. L. Wu, H. R. Lu, Y. Chen, N. S. Xia, T. S. P. Naipospos, K. Y. Yuen, S. S. Hassan, S. Bahri, T. D. Nguyen, R. G. Webster, J. S. M. Peiris, and Y. Guan, "Establishment of Multiple Sublineages of H5N1 Influenza Virus in Asia: Implications for Pandemic Control," *PNAS* 103, no. 8 (February 10, 2006): 2,845–50.

[50] Vaclav Smil, *Global Catastrophes and Trends: The Next Fifty Years* (MIT Press).

[51] William Gates, "The Next Outbreak? We're Not Ready," TED, https://youtu.be/6Af6b wyiwI.

ferret to another as a droplet-transmitted infection.[52] The virus was now airborne! The firestorm of debate that followed had proponents hailing the merits of such work in furtherance of mankind's understanding of virulence, transmissibility, and the fundamental determinants of immune resistance and vaccinology while opponents were aghast at the potential hazards of such research regarding accidental mutagenesis that could easily run amuck and unleash a global biologic catastrophe. [53, 54]

Moratorium on Doomsday

The growing drumbeat of such concerns, in 2014, led a group of scientists in Cambridge, Massachusetts to form the Cambridge Working Group (CWG) to push for a moratorium and tighter regulation on all potentially hazardous biologic research involving organisms of pandemic potential.

---

[52] M. Imai, T. Watanabe, M. Hatta, S. C. Das, M. Ozawa, K. Shinya, G. Zhong, A. Hanson, H. Katsura, S. Watanabe, C. Li, E. Kawakami, S. Yamada, M. Kiso, Y. Suzuki, E. A. Maher, G. Neumann, and Y. Kawaoka, "Experimental Adaptation of an Influenza H5 HA Confers Respiratory Droplet Transmission to a Reassortant H5 HA/H1N1 Virus in Ferrets," *Nature* 496, no. 7,403 (May 2, 2012): 420–8, doi: 10.1038/nature10831, PMID: 22722205; PMCID: PMC3388103; E. J. Schrauwen, S. Herfst, L. M. Leijten, P. van Run, T. M. Bestebroer, M. Linster, R. Bodewes, J. H. Kreijtz, G. F. Rimmelzwaan, A. D. Osterhaus, R. A. Fouchier, T. Kuiken, and D. van Riel, "The Multibasic Cleavage Site in H5N1 Virus Is Critical for Systemic Spread along the Olfactory and Hematogenous Routes in Ferrets," *J Virol* 86, no. 7 (April 2012): 3,975–84, doi: 10.1128/JVI.06828-11, epub January 25, 2012, PMID: 22278228, PMCID: PMC3302532.

[53] Barbara Holzer, Sophie B. Morgan, Yumi Matsuoka, Matthew Edmans, Francisco J. Salguero, Helen Everett, Sharon M. Brookes, Emily Porter, Ronan MacLoughlin, Bryan Charleston, Kanta Subbarao, Alain Townsend, and Elma Tchilian, "Comparison of Heterosubtypic Protection in Ferrets and Pigs Induced by a Single-Cycle Influenza Vaccine," *J Immunol* 200, no. 12 (June 15, 2018): 4,068–77.

[54] M. Lipsitch, "Why Do Exceptionally Dangerous Gain-of-Function Experiments in Influenza?" in *Influenza Virus: Methods in Molecular Biology*, ed. Y. Yamauchi, vol. 1,836 (New York: Humana Press, 2018), https://doi.org/10.1007/978-1-4939-8678-1_29.

The push by CWG was given greater urgency since it coincided with a series of unintentional lapses in laboratory safety at the CDC, FDA and USDA involving anthrax bacteria, samples of smallpox virus and H9N2 and H5N1 influenza strains.[55] The July 14, 2014, moratorium call on all research involving pathogens of pandemic potential, by the 18 member CWG which was endorsed by over three hundred scientists, academics, and physicians was ultimately followed by a decision of the White House Office of Science and Technology and the Department of Health and Human Services to institute a gain of function research and funding moratorium that lasted from 2014 until 2017.[56]

The world owes much of the ensuing evidence to the investigative work performed by members of the private group DRASTIC which is an acronym for Decentralized Radical Autonomous Search Team Investigating Covid-19. This group of globally widespread internet sleuths have managed to sleuth out and excavate a huge trove of diverse data that has enabled much of the world's policy bodies to penetrate the obfuscating wall of institutional obstructionism surrounding this pandemic. Widely acclaimed by agencies and news organizations as doing higher quality work than governments, some notable contributors in this effort both within and without the DRASTIC team include Gilles Demaneuf, William Bostickson, Prasanjeet Ray (aka The Seeker), Monali Rahalkar and investigative journalists of the Wall Street Journal.

---

[55] CDC Newsroom, CDC Releases After-Action Report on Recent Anthrax Incident, Highlights Steps to Improve Laboratory Quality and Safety, CDC Website, https://www.cdc.gov/media/releases/2014/p0711-lab-safety.html (anthrax); Jocelyn Kaiser, "Six Vials of Smallpox Discovered in U.S. Lab," July 8, 2014, https://www.science.org/content/article/six-vials-smallpox-discovered-us-lab (smallpox); and Jocelyn Kaiser, "Scientists Call for limits on Creating Dangerous Pathogens, July 158, 2014, https://www.science.org/content/article/scientists-call-limit-creating-dangerous-pathogens (H5N1-contaminated H9N2).

[56] J. l. Husbands, "The Challenge of FRAMING for efforts to Mitigate the Risks of 'Dual Use' Research in the Life Sciences," *Futures* 102 (September 2018): 104–13; Marc Lipsitch, Kevin Esvelt, and Thomas Inglesby, "Calls for Caution in Genome Engineering Should Be a Model for Similar Dialogue on Pandemic Pathogen Research," *Annals of Internal Medicine*, November 17, 2015.

EcoHealth and NIH

EcoHealth Alliance was created by Peter Daszak, a conservation biologist, in 2011 to foster a scientific and environmental alliance to understand the delicate balance between ecological health, its degradation, wildlife health, and human health. Daszak felt the combination of global warming, ecological degradation, and global freshwater crisis was increasing the probability for outbreaks of new diseases. It is well recognized that there currently exist many animal and plant microbes and viruses' humans never encounter because human populations do not have significant contact with these wilderness flora and fauna. But Daszak saw ecological degradation, climate change, and freshwater decline as a trifecta of conditions creating a perfect storm for the emergence of new diseases. He argued that these conditions were reducing agricultural harvesting of protein, increasing contact between wild animals and humans, and pushing increased exposures due to pressure on human populations that were already under nutritional pressure. He felt that scientists were too siloed in their narrow disciplines. EcoHealth Alliance was conceived as an organization that would bring microbiologists, virologists, epidemiologists, climatologists, soil-science experts, agricultural experts, botanists, and zoologists in a cross-disciplinary network to study and map out the risks, as well as guide the development of visionary policies by governmental agencies.

It would seem inconceivable that such an organization would find itself in the eye of the firestorm surrounding the origins of SARS-CoV-2. On May 27, 2014, EcoHealth Alliance was awarded a $4.3 million RO1 grant (# **R01AI110964**) to fund research towards "Understanding the Risk of Bat Coronavirus Emergence"[57]. The research proposed to study bat coronaviruses of the type that caused the first SARS epidemic of 2003.[58] The original award was to run from 2014 in annual renewal

---

[57] https://www.usaspending.gov/award/ASST_NON_R01AI110964_7529

[58] Understanding the risk of bat coronavirus emergence. Sept. 8, 2021. https://theintercept.com/document/2021/09/08/understanding-the-risk-of-bat-coronavirus-emergence/.

increments till June 2023. As fate would have it the grant was not renewed after June 2019 after about $3.7 million dollars had been spent for reasons that will become evident. The Ecohealth grant was issued prior to the October 2014 NIH funding pause on all new pandemic-related research, and hence, NIH Grant # **R01AI110964** slipped under the regulatory oversight radar and continued to operate. In addition, the wording of the grant research proposal was merely to identify the prevalence of coronaviruses in bat populations and to catalogue the possibility of an emergence. This stated aim appeared on surface innocuous enough to slip beneath the regulatory oversight radar that existed at the time. To make things more convenient, the grant was to be carried out overseas in the Wuhan Institute of Virology in collaboration with Daszak's long-time collaborator Shi Zhengli who had long studied the type of bats that harbored SARS-type coronaviruses and was famous in China as the "batwoman". These bat species (Rhinolophidae) that were the natural reservoir of these coronaviruses were residents of the cave systems in the mountains of Enshi prefecture in the Hubei province of China. Under the terms of the collaboration drafted, EcoHealth used some of the NIH funds to execute the research at WIV using WIV resources with EcoHealth being the grant prime recipient and the WIV as a sub-recipient. Daszak's scientific relationship with Shi Zhengli, a WIV virologist, goes back to 2006, and the two have coauthored many papers on SARS-type bat coronaviruses. Another significant collaborator on the same project was Ralph Baric of the University of North Carolina, Chapel Hill whose humanized mice bearing the human ACE-2 receptor would serve as an animal model to test the infectivity of SARS-type coronaviruses in the later years of the grant.

THE BASIS OF R01 AI110964

Scientists do not submit grant proposals without knowing to some degree beforehand the answers to the questions they want to ask. Contrary to popular belief scientists do not ask for funding and then go out into the wilderness to conduct their research. Often what they want to study has already been studied by them to some degree and this forms the basis of the funding proposal. Both Daszak and Shi Zhengli already knew in 2014 that a certain cave in South China harbored bats that were capable of sickening humans with a respiratory illnessbut did not reveal this information in RO1 A1110964 grant proposal.

In 2020, Prasanjeet Ray of the DRASTIC team researching internet records of scientific publication on SARS-type infections in China unearthed a masters and doctoral thesis of a Chinese student. The thesis which was published in Chinese upon translation, revealed that in April 2012 six miners harvesting bat guano from a defunct copper mine near Tong Guan in Mojiang Hani county of the Yunnan province fell ill with a mysterious and serious respiratory illness[59],[60],[61] . Three of the six miners would eventually die. Biological samples from these patients were tested at the WIV and were positive for a SARS-type virus infection in at least 2 out of the 6 cases.

Shi Zhengli proceeded to visit the Tong Guan mine in 2013 and collected at least 9 novel virus samples. An October 2013 paper coauthored by her and Daszak in Nature announces the discovery of 2 novel bat coronaviruses isolated from the Chinese horseshoe bat species which she labeled as RsSHCO14 and Rs3367, Shi also announced the successful laboratory culture of a bat coronavirus strain that bore 99.9% identity with Rs3367 and therefore presumably was derived from the Rs3367 wildtype parent. This lab strain was given the name bat-SL-CoV-WIV1 and was found to infect human cells, civets, and bats via the ACE-2 receptor. Shi goes on to assert that "Our results provide the strongest evidence to date that Chinese horseshoe bats are natural reservoirs of SARS-CoV and that intermediate hosts may not be necessary for direct human infection by some bat SL-CoVs. They also highlight the importance of pathogen-discovery programs targeting

---

[59] https://drive.google.com/file/d/1_Md2GVJvMDbsNzS8X2wbTvxgCerK9Qsn/view

[60] https://drive.google.com/file/d/1OdWCjEJEqEyxbujWwvkf0hknxDoRTCAw/view

[61] Demaneuf, G: https://gillesdemaneuf.medium.com/wiv-ecohealth-the-mojiang-miners-cases-and-a-bat-sampling-trip-in-april-2012-74be5c2e0a0a

high-risk wildlife groups in emerging disease hotspots as a strategy for pandemic preparedness"[62].

PRE-ADAPTATION TO HUMAN SPREAD

The finding by the WIV scientists as detailed in the October 2013 Nature paper of bat coronavirus strains in the wild capable of direct transmission to humans without an intermediary animal host is important because what follows is that WIV and EcoHealth's subsequent work was all concerning derivatives of this progenitor bat virus strain. One of the first observations of epidemiologists and virologists in Dec2019 and Jan 2020 was that SARS-CoV2 was not behaving as if it were a virus freshly entering the human population for the first time. Most viruses that jump from animals to humans go through a period of host adaptation. It is like a dating game between a boy and a girl pairing up for the first time. The initial interactions are tentative as the virus evolves towards its best fit to its host. So, in such cases, the initial spread is hesitant and sporadic. By contrast, the COVID-19 illness produced by SARS-CoV2 was spreading like wildfire in November and December 2019. The initial R_0 of the virus in November and December 2019 (R_0 is a co-efficient of its transmissibility and virulence) was estimated at 2.5 to 4.0, with some estimates of as high as 6.5. Essentially a R_0 of 3 means that each infected individual would infect three additional individuals before the disease ran its course in that person. To provide some perspective Ebola has a R_0 of 1.5. The SARS-CoV2 virus was behaving as if, it was already well adapted to its human host. Such a situation would be true under two scenarios. 1) SARS-CoV2 was already circulating at low levels in the human population for some time prior to 2019. But apart from the 6 cases of the Tong Guan miner's illness there was no evidence of SARS-like illness between 2013 to September 2019. In addition, the level of exposure of the miners in the Tong Guan cave to

---

[62] Ge, XY., Li, JL., Yang, XL. *et al.* Isolation and characterization of a bat SARS-like coronavirus that uses the ACE2 receptor. *Nature* **503**, 535–538 (2013). https://doi.org/10.1038/nature12711

bat genetic material through contact with bat excreta and inhaled particles within the closed environment of the mine's narrow passages at depths of up to 150 feet, ensured that the infective inoculum that these 6 patients experienced would have been extremely high. That spoke to an initial wild-type strain with a low virulence and transmissibility. This would explain the scenario of a lack of other cases in the 7 years after April 20121, where the bat viruses with human infective capability would have existed in that region, but the virus would not readily spread spontaneously into the human population on a random casual contact, and would instead require high concentrated exposure to the virus. 2) The SARS-CoV2 was a human-capable bat virus, to begin with that had subsequently acquired an enhancement of its virulence capability that enabled its wildfire spread once it got the opportunity to infect even 1 or 2 individuals. But how did that happen? To investigate that we must turn back the pages of events by a few years.

A UNIQUE BREED

Scientists are a unique breed of individuals. In addition to exceptionally high levels of intelligence, and analytic and deductive logic, collectively they exhibit personality traits of unbridled curiosity, innovative thinking, a willingness to boldly test boundaries and to design methods and tools to further this thirst for satisfaction of their intellectual hunger. For the most part, the scientific community is also possessed of high indices of integrity and a moral code of beneficence to humanity. But this code of beneficence is always in juxtaposition and in some respects subservient to the end goal of all scientists' endeavors, which is to continually satisfy their intellectual curiosity. The means of achievement of that end goal is based on employing the tools of their intellect and a willingness to push boundaries. The events that followed the 2014 moratorium on the gain of function research must be viewed in this context of the innate tendency towards intellectual hubris of the scientific community in general. The three years that followed the CWG moratorium in 2014 were always suffered by the scientific community as a burden and resented by many as shackles on research that many virologists felt was overzealous regulatory oversight. The power of the pharmaceutical-academic-regulatory complex is immense. So, when the Trump administration arrived with its philosophy of dismantling regulation at every level and unleashing the hounds of business and enterprise, the scientific community felt their time had come. In 2017 a group of thirty-seven scientists formed Scientists for Science and pushed for a resumption of research on dangerous pathogens arguing that such research was essential and that adequate safety measures existed to protect the public. [63,64] This argument found a receptive ear with the Trump administration and in December 2017, the NIH resumed funding of gain-of-function research on pathogens of pandemic potential. [65]

GOFR and DURC

One of the key issues of debate is how to define what constitutes gain-of-function research (GOFR or "gopher"). GOFR may be defined based on (a) the design of the actual experiment or (b) the express intent of the experiment. For example, a GOFR experiment may be designed to specifically introduce a mutation in a microbial (bacteria or virus) genome to confer a new property the original organism (wild type) did not have. Even though the new function does not increase the organism's virulence or pathogenicity, this would be classified as GOFR since there is a new function acquired.

An alternate example of GOFR would be the repeated manual passaging (exposure) of a microbe to a whole animal or animal cells in

---

[63] A. Edelmann, J. Moody, and R. Light, "Disparate Foundations of Scientists' Policy Positions on Contentious Biomedical Research," *Proc Natl Acad Sci U S A* 114, no. 24 (June 2017): 6,262–67.

[64] W. P. Duprex, R. A, Fouchier, M. J. Imperiale, M. Lipsitch, and D. A. Relman, "Gain-of-Function Experiments: Time for a Real Debate," *Nat Rev Microbiol.* 13, no. 1 (January 2015): 58–64.

[65] Francis S. Collins, "NIH Lifts Funding Pause on Gain-of-Function Research," *National Institutes of Health*, December 19, 2017.

culture not a normal host of the organism to allow the acquisition by the organism of the ability to replicate and thrive in the new non-native cell or animal. Here, the intent is specific acquisition of extra-species infectivity and propagability by a microbe that hitherto would never have infected this new animal or cell.

It is this gray zone of potential interpretation of GOFR that makes the regulation of GOFR tricky. For example, a property like increased pathogenicity, transmissibility, and virulence may be a multistep process. A GOFR experiment may result in acquisition of a new nonpathogenic, nonvirulence function, but this new function can be a link in the chain, where the next step would be the acquisition of increased virulence and lethality. In this manner, the ball is tipped a little closer to the edge of chaos.

This is very well seen even in the SARS-CoV-2 pandemic. The original wild type of virus prevalent from November 2019 till April 2020 spontaneously mutated into alpha, beta, gamma, delta, and omicron variants with progressive increase in transmissibility. From a mechanistic perspective, each variant was becoming progressively better adapted to transmission, replication, and propagation in the human population. This, in certain respects, is nature performing GOFR, except it's occurring as random chance over a huge number of iterative attempts.

So, when a government functionary declares to a congressional committee that its agency has never funded GOFR at any lab or research institution, the statement could be technically truthful but not really accurate on the basis of how GOFR is being defined.

Due to the inherent difficulties of the definition of what constitutes GOFR, research on pathogens with potential for accidental release or potential for intentional release was classified as "dual use research of concern" (DURC) requiring additional regulatory and institutional oversight.[66,67] With the onset of the COVID-19 pandemic, critics

---

[66] United States Government Policy for Oversight of Life Sciences DURC. https://www.phe.gov/s3/dualuse/Pages/USGOversightPolicy.aspx

[67] Dual Use Research of Concern (DURC) Institutional Review Entity. https://oir.nih.gov/sourcebook/committees-advisory-ddir/dual-use-research-concern-durc-institutional-review-entity

of GOFR have been vociferous in emphasizing that the enhanced classification DURC should have been necessarily instituted on all bat virus research, even if the projects did not constitute actual GOFR manipulation of the viruses so isolated.[68]

DARPA DEFUSE PROJECT

In April 2018 EcoHealth submitted a $14 million multi-year bat coronavirus research proposal called DEFUSE that outlined its plans to isolate the viruses from the Tong Guan cave complex, and engage in genetic recombination and GOFR research on these samples at the WIV. The researchers planned to create chimeric bat viruses and immunologically reactive spike protein vaccine conjugates that they proposed to reintroduce into wild free bat populations in the same Tong Guan cave system in a massive bat anti-SARS vaccination program. The intent was to carry out a genetic modification and immunological modification program of unprecedented scale and scope. DARPA rejected the DEFUSE research proposal in December 2018 because they deemed it too risky and because the proposal lacked appropriate safeguards for GOFR-DURC capable research[69]. Though the grant funding was turned down in its entirety, the DEFUSE proposal is alarming in its stated intentions. Once again, the existence of this rejected proposal would never have seen the light of day except for the work of the DRASTIC team who unearthed the evidence in the course of sleuthing for answers to the COVID origins debate[70]. The experiments outlined in the DEFUSE proposal is a rare look into the thought process of the virologists at EcoHealth, the WIV and its collaborating institutions and

---

[68] N. Shinomiya, J. Minari, G. Yoshizawa, M. Dando, and L. Shang, "Reconsidering the Need for Gain-of-Function Research on Enhanced Potential Pandemic Pathogens in the Post-COVID-19 Era," *Front Bioeng Biotechnol.* 10 (August 26, 2022): 966,586.
[69] https://www.documentcloud.org/documents/21066966-defuse-proposal
[70] https://drasticresearch.org/2021/09/21/the-defuse-project-documents/

raise serious long-term concerns about the continuing risk of pandemic grade research to humanity in our world today.

The concerns raised in the DEFUSE proposal belong to 4 categories.

1) **GOFR Experiments:** The proposal detailed virulence-enhancing experiments that were proposed to be done on the Tong Guan mine bat viruses that already were capable of binding to human ACE-2 receptors and infecting human cells. The DEFUSE proposal planned to insert a Furin Cleavage Site (FCS) into the SARS-CoV spike protein structure. An FCS has long been recognized as a virulence-enhancing mutation in many viruses and as such the SARS-type coronaviruses do not commonly bear an FCS in their structure, though it is seen in other lineages of coronaviruses. As I mentioned earlier, scientists seldom write a grant detailing an experiment that they have not at least already attempted in a preliminary manner to ensure that they would be successful in the attempt. So the evidence of this intent reveals that the EcoHealth-WIV researchers were (a) thinking of ways to enhance the virulence of the human pathogenic bat coronaviruses they had harvested from the Tong Guan mine, and, (b) in all probability had already created a variant with precisely such an inserted FCS in the spike protein. IT is also evident from the wording that the researchers knew that their viruses were already capable of infecting human cells and already possessed at least epidemic causing capability.. ""However, our test cave site in Yunnan Province, harbors a quasispecies (QS) population assemblage that contains all the genetic components of epidemic SARS-CoV . We have isolated three strains there (WIV1, WIV16 and SHCO14) that unlike other SARSr-CoVs, do not contain two deletions in the receptor-binding domain (RBD) of the spike, have far higher sequence identity to SARS-CoV (Fig. 1), use human ACE2 receptor for cell entry, as SARS-CoV does (Fig. 2), and replicate efficiently in various animal and human cells."

2) **DURC conflicts:** Grant monies were intended to pay WIV researcher's salaries at least in part. It is relevant the WIV is at least partly a Chinese military lab and conducts classified bioweapons work for the PLA in addition to non-classified cilian research. The idea of seeking US military agency funding of research with GOFR/DURC parameters in collaboration with a foreign governmental laboratory with military ties is alarming, to say the least. It is also evident that the researchers attempted to minimize this by including language that attempted to bypass P3CO (GOFR) and DURC framework restrictions by asserting that such risks did not exist, thereby demonstrating that the grant authors were not unaware of these conflicts.

3) **Poorly Regulated Wild Population Biologic modification:** EcoHealth planned to conduct regular field visits to the Tong Guan cave to collect bat samples and to inoculate wild free-ranging bats with lab-engineered anti-SARSCoV vaccines in order to eradicate these viral strains in the bats themselves. The proposal offered no discussion of the existing level of understanding of the bat immune system and what could be the possible ecological ramifications of such unrestricted modifications of a wild free-ranging flying mammal population.

4) **Unregulated Transport of Infective Viral strains across international borders:** EcoHealth proposed to ship viral samples overseas to collaborating investigators in UNC Chapel Hill and to Duke Universities Singapore campus for additional work. "Samples will be preserved in viral transport medium, immediately frozen in liquid nitrogen dry shippers, and transported to partner laboratories with a maintained cold chain and under strict biosafety protocols." They also assert that "Drs Shi, Zhang, and Daszak have collaborated together since 2002 and have been involved in running joint conferences, and shipping samples into and out of China."[71]. This piece of evidence raises the question as to how many SARS strains are

[71] https://www.documentcloud.org/documents/21066966-defuse-proposal

already floating in the US in the repositories of laboratories at UNC Chapel Hill and other institutions and what is the level of oversight on these. The researchers also claimed that EcoHealth and its collaborating labs in China, Singapore, and the US already have more than 180 SARS strains that have not yet been examined for spill-over potential, and that work on these strains would also be carried out in the laboratories of collaborating institutions in these countries.

On a scale of just scope and audacity the DEFUSE proposal is an example of a staggeringly risky endeavor. It is now well documented by multiple sources that Chinese researchers often entered these caves without appropriate PPE and handled bats in the field and in the lab in BSL-2 level biosafety environments. A BSL-2 level at its best is comparable to a researcher working with a surgical mask, gloves and lab coat in a laminar flow hood that is vented without filtration of its outflow. At its worst, a BSL-2 would be no more than what exists in a dentist's office. Though DARPA rejected this proposal citing biosafety and biosecurity concerns, the fact that these researchers saw fit to submit such a proposal reveals the operational culture of their research conditions and their own thought process of what these researchers would consider safe and responsible research.

Natural Emergence or Lab Leak

The question of the precise origin of the SARS-CoV-2 virus and the pandemic it caused is still far from settled. The official consensus has so far been that the SARS-CoV-2 virus and the COVID-19 pandemic was the outcome of a natural spillover from bats to humans arising from proximity of each in the unsanitary wet market conditions of the Wuhan animal market. But ever since the early days, there have remained whispers of its origin as a lab leak from the Wuhan Institute of Virology. The fact that the grant conditions and oversight exercised by the NIH on the grant awarded to EcoHealth Alliance and its collaborator, Wuhan

Institute of Virology, had serious deficiencies in regulatory oversight is one of the factors cited by proponents of this view.

In addition, the lack of transparency afforded by Chinese authorities to investigative teams attempting to determine the pandemic origins has not helped settle the debate either. Investigators from the United States, Europe, and the WHO have repeatedly decried the Chinese government's refusal to make available critical data that could help resolve key issues in the COVID-19 origins debate. The geopolitical ramifications of these investigations into the origins of a pandemic that has caused 25 million dead and nearly $9 trillion in global economic loss are astronomical, and hence, the barriers raised by the Chinese government are not entirely surprising. Despite all that, the official view that COVID-19 "most probably" arose as a natural spillover event in the environment of the Wuhan wet market, even though it cannot be conclusively eliminated that it did not occur as an accidental leak from the WIV lab because of a lapse in biosafety protocols has recently come under serious challenge.

While multiple investigations by WHO teams and other teams into WIV as a potential source of COVID-19 have failed to establish a definitive link, it is now accepted that WIV did harvest bat species that harbored coronavirus strains closely related to SARS-CoV-2 that emerged in Wuhan. In addition, WIV did engage in experiments from June 2018 to June 2019, in which an engineered version of a bat coronavirus expressing SARS spike proteins was evaluated on transgenic mice expressing human ACE2 receptor. EcoHealth Alliance's own final report to NIH from a section labeled "In vivo infection of Human ACE2 (hACE2) expression mice with SARSr-CoV S protein variants in year 5" is alarming to say the least. [72]

Essentially the WIV/EcoHealth scientists created an animal model of transgenic mice that had been engineered to express the human ACE2 receptor on their cell surfaces. The WIV scientists took four different strains of recombinant bat SARS-CoV viral strains created by grafting

---

[72] Understanding the risk of bat coronavirus emergence. https://oversight.house.gov/wp-content/uploads/2021/10/Year-5-EHAv.pdf.

different pieces of the Spike protein (S protein). While 3 of the 4 strains had only 50% mortality, the 4th chimeric virus killed 6 out of 8 mice infected and the viral titers steadily increased as the days post infection increased until the viral load reached more than 10^9 genome copies/g at the demise point of the mouse. Autopsy and histopathological section examination revealed gross tissue lesions and lymphocyte infiltration in the lung which was maximal in the mice infected with the rWIV1-SHC014 S strain suggesting that the pathogenicity of SHC014 is higher than other tested bat SARSr-CoVs strains. The viral load of the chimeric rWIV1-SHCO14 strain-infected mice at the time of death was a staggering 1 billion genome copies per gram of mouse brain tissue, whereas three other chimeric viruses (rWIV1, rWIV1-WIV15S, and rWIV1-4231S) were undetectable in mice tissue by day four after infection.

Strikingly, the NIH deemed this experiment not a GOFR since the original viruses being studied were not viruses that were pathogenic to humans, a determination that is hotly contested by other virologists. Several virologists have called the relationship between the NIH and EcoHealth unduly cozy and point to a lack of true regulatory oversight and accountability.[73] Indeed, a review of all the data emerging in this saga strongly implies the parties may have done the equivalent of a wink and a nod to allow scientists to skate at the far edge of the boundaries of what could be defined as not GOFR or DURC in an effort to push the boundaries of zoonotic biology knowledge.[74]

---

[73] Sharon Lerner, Mara Hvistendahl, Maia Hibbett. The Intercept. Sept. 9, 2021. NIH documents provide new evidence U.S. funded Gain-of-Function research in Wuhan. https://theintercept.com/2021/09/09/covid-origins-gain-of-function-research/.

[74] Sharon Lerner, Mara Hvistendahl. The Intercept. Nov. 3, 2021. NIH officials worked with Ecohealth Alliance to evade restrictions on coronavirus experiments. https://theintercept.com/2021/11/03/coronavirus-research-ecohealth-nih-emails/.

SEPTEMBER 2019

A series a strange events in early September 2019 in the city of Wuhan point to a mysterious convergence of facts indicating that the pandemic may have arisen as a lab leak event at the WIV. Early reports suggested that three researchers from the Wuhan Institute of Virology (WIV) had fallen ill with a respiratory illness of sufficient severity to be hospitalized in September 2019.[75] These illnesses would predate the first reported COVID cases in China by more than a month. The intelligence reported was derived from multiple sources and was described as of "exquisite quality" and very "precise." These reports at the time were met with vehement rebuttals from the Chinese government and even from Western scientists who praised the scientific integrity of Dr. Shi Zhengli, who ran the coronavirus lab at WIV and who was the collaborator with EcoHealth Alliance on the NIH-funded SARS chimeric virus project described earlier. Dr. Zhengli's work has been variously described by fellow scientists as very important and of the highest quality. But it must be noted that Dali Yang in a March 2020 report in the Washington Post detailed the Chinese government's penchant for coverup of viral outbreaks, intimidation of whistleblowers and obfuscation [76],

On September 12, 2019, the WIV viral database repository of the gene sequences of every virus ever harvested or studied at WIV, that until then had been a publicly accessible resource for scientists worldwide, suddenly and inexplicably went dark. Chinese authorities initially claimed that a massive server upgrade was being performed. Later the reason was modified to allegations that they were being hacked. To this date the WIV database has not come online. On the heels of this event, WIV was placed under the administrative command of Chinese military

---

[75] Michael R. Gordon, Warren P. Strobel and Drew Hinshaw. Wall Street Journal May 23, 2021. Intelligence on sick staff at Wuhan lab fuels debate on Covid-19 origin. https://www.wsj.com/articles/intelligence-on-sick-staff-at-wuhan-lab-fuels-debate-on-covid-19-origin-11621796228

[76] Dali L. Yang, "Wuhan Officials Tried to Cover up COVID-19—and Sent It Careening Outward," *The Washington Post*, March 10, 2020.

general. Lastly in the same month, an outside air-conditioning and ventilation contractor was brought in to perform a massive $606 million overhaul of WIV air handling and ventilation systems[77]. These findings were part of an 84-page memo released to the US House Foreign Affairs Committee in August 2021.

Despite all this, the question of a lab leak essentially has foundered on the shoals of noncooperation by the Chinese authorities, who have, to this date, denied investigative teams access to key environmental data, biological samples, lab safety data, and other records from WIV and the Wuhan town from the earliest days of the pandemic. This fact was reiterated by FBI Director Wray who observed that the Chinese government has been doing its utmost to thwart and obstruct the work of US and other international agencies. [78]

It is now unofficially maintained by most scientists and nearly all US government agencies that the pandemic arose as an unintentional lab leak event due to a failure of biosafety protocols and practices in the WIV. It is widely accepted off the record that the researchers at WIV were engaged in GOFR research on human infection capable bat SARS-type coronaviruses with a high probability of virulence enhancement of the wild-type virus by introduction of a Furin Cleavage site. This coupled with the fact that these experiments were being performed in BSL-2 grade facilities with inadequate ventilation may have resulted in infection of one or more lab personnel who may have spread the virus elsewhere in the city. This event was aggressively suppressed by the Chinese government in the period from the end of August 2019 till January 2020 a behavior that is consistent with the Chinese government's penchant for coverup of viral outbreaks, intimidation of whistleblowers, and obfuscation [79].

---

[77] https://www.nationalreview.com/news/wuhan-lab-air-circulation-systems-were-defective-ahead-of-first-known-covid-cases-congressional-report-finds/

[78] Adam Sabes. Fox News March 1, 2023. FBI Director says Covid pandemic 'most likely' originated from Chinese lab. https://www.foxnews.com/politics/fbi-director-says-covid-pandemic-most-likely-originated-chinese-lab

[79] Dali L. Yang, "Wuhan Officials Tried to Cover up COVID-19—and Sent It Careening Outward," The Washington Post, March 10, 2020.

The fact that the research activities at the WIV had been at least partly funded by the US Government through the NIH is source of embarrassment to both Republican and Democrat sides of the aisle resulting in at least some reluctance to have an open dialogue into these mishaps. The situation was even more bluntly stated by Dr. Marty Makary, MD, MPH, at the House Select Subcommittee on the Coronavirus Pandemic on February 28, 2023. In forcefully direct testimony Dr Makary argued that the only reason that a debate existed over the origins of the pandemic is because of the embarrassing fact that the U.S. had funded bat coronavirus research in a high-level Chinese virology lab that was 5 miles away from the epicenter of the pandemic outbreak. He called it a no-brainer and said that any attempt to acquire more information would only confirm a lab leak as the source. [80]

But since January 2023, a series of disparate events have begun to point toward a quiet undercurrent of opinion in the US administration that new thinking on pandemic research and pandemic preparedness must prevail.. The first of these events was a little-publicized report that was released on January 27, 2023. The National Science Advisory Board for Biosecurity (NSABB) issued a draft report titled, *Proposed Biosecurity Oversight Framework for the Future of Science* with its latest recommendations on the subject of GOFR, Potential Pandemic Pathogen Care and Oversight (P3CO), and DURC.[81] The report has recommended broadening the rules that determine whether proposed

---

[80] MedPage Today Mar 1, 2023. Hopkins' Makary tells lawmakers COVID lab leak a No brainer. https://www.medpagetoday.com/infectiousdisease/covid19/103341

[81] Jocelyn Kaiser. Science. Jan 20, 2023. U.S. should expand rules for risky virus research to more pathogens, panel says. https://www.science.org/content/article/u-s-should-expand-rules-risky-virus-research-more-pathogens-panel-says

studies count as dual-use research to include work with all human, plant, and animal pathogens, even those causing only mild disease.[82, 83]

Then on February 10, 2023, a group of scientists announced the formation of a nonprofit organization called Protect Our Future to advocate for tighter biolab safety and to prevent "lab-generated pandemics that could threaten the survival of the human species." [84] Separately there was the public admission by FBI Director Christopher Wray in a Fox News interview on February 28, 2023, that the FBI had revised its assessment to come to the conclusion that the pandemic most likely arose as the result of a "lab incident" in Wuhan. [85] Director Wray observed that the issue at hand concerned the leak of a deadly pathogen from a Chinese government lab.

Director Wray's statement represented the first official and significant escalation from the FBI's prior assessment in 2021 that the bureau had only a "moderate confidence" in the lab leak theory.

The FBI assessment also represented the second US governmental agency to assert that the pandemic may have originated because of a breakdown in biosafety protocols. At around the same time as the FBI's reassessment, the US Energy Department released a new assessment that the pandemic originated because of an accidental lab leak from a Chinese virology lab. Like the FBI, the energy department's assessment was also a reversal from its previous opinion on the matter and was part

---

[82] Proposed biosecurity oversight framework for the future of science. https://osp.od.nih.gov/wp-content/uploads/2023/01/DRAFT-NSABB-WG-Report.pdf; https://www.nih.gov/about-nih/who-we-are/nih-director/statements/statement-report-national-science-advisory-board-biosecurity;

[83] Jocelyn Kaiser. Science Jan 30, 2023. U.S. Scientists brace for tighter scrutiny of potentially risky research. https://www.science.org/content/article/u-s-scientists-brace-tighter-scrutiny-potentially-risky-research

[84] Jocelyn Kaiser. Science Feb. 6, 2023. Critics of risky virus studies launch nonprofit to push for research halt, tighter safety rules. https://www.science.org/content/article/critics-risky-virus-studies-launch-nonprofit-push-research-halt-tighter-safety-rules

[85] Adam Sabes. Fox News March 1, 2023. FBI Director says Covid pandemic 'most likely' originated from Chinese lab. https://www.foxnews.com/politics/fbi-director-says-covid-pandemic-most-likely-originated-chinese-lab

of a classified intelligence report provided to the White House and select members of Congress and this was reported by the Wall Street Journal.[86]

The question of the pandemic's origins is not one of political blame and shame gaming. It is imperative for humanity to understand how the greatest biological catastrophe of this century came about so we may be better able to forestall a future occurrence. The pandemic so far has resulted in measurable global monetary damage of at least $8.5 trillion and counting. The immeasurable damages are far higher by several orders of magnitude. If you begin to count the nearly 25 million lives lost, the millions of lives impaired by long COVID, the millions of children orphaned globally by loss of one or both parents, the millions of orphan minors consumed by human trafficking, the educational development lost, the generational wisdom lost by the mortality of seniors, the cost becomes incalculable. The search for answers is, therefore, not likely to cease any time soon, and neither should it ever if we as a species are to avoid becoming a victim of our own hubris.

---

[86] Michael R. Gordon, Warren P. Strobel. Wall Street Journal Feb 26, 2023. Lab leak most likely origin of Covid-19 pandemic, Energy department now says. https://www.wsj.com/articles/covid-origin-china-lab-leak-807b7b0a

CHAPTER 7

Kali's Dance

Now I am become Death the destroyer of worlds.
—Robert Oppenheimer paraphrasing the Bhagavad
Gita on witnessing the detonation of the atomic bomb

The Reaper's Domain

March 27, 2020

I got a call from the director of nursing at an Alzheimer's and memory care facility where I was a visiting physician. Some of her residents were showing respiratory symptoms. Would I be able to come and test them? My nurse and I put together a COVID travel kit consisting of PPE, disinfecting supplies, testing supplies, and laboratory forms. I already knew that approaching a confused patient with dementia dressed like an astronaut in a hazmat suit was not likely to go well, and I warned my nurse to ready for agitation and possible violence.

This was no small matter at that time. We were dealing with a lethal respiratory pathogen against which we had no immunity and no treatment. The patients who we were planning to test were likely to fight, kick, and punch us as we tried to swab their nasal secretions. Apart from the prospect of physical injury, the possibility of exposure to infected material was very high.

In addition, this was not the same as testing in our parking lot in a controlled environment with infected patients inside their own vehicles and only our arms entering their space. In an Alzheimer's facility, it is impossible to have an infected person maintain a six-foot distance or even comprehend that they must remain in isolation. In such a place, confused and sick individuals would be wandering everywhere in the corridors, sneezing, and coughing and wiping hands smeared with runny nasal secretions everywhere. We were entering the reaper's domain, swimming in a sea of infective viral particles.

We reached the facility and set up our gowning station outside in the parking lot beside our vehicle. Armed with our supplies, we walked into the facility. What we saw there was an infectious disease nightmare. About a dozen confused seniors were wandering the corridor sneezing and coughing. None of the patients in the facility were masked. Residents were clustered at tables in the dining room, and a maskless nursing aide was conducting a group exercise.

I tested eight residents and two staff members. All were positive. The following week, we returned and tested all the staff and more residents who were symptomatic. Several staff and all symptomatic residents were positive. In addition, I noted that several of the staff worked additional shifts at other nursing home facilities. This meant that there was a free flow of infected individuals between these facilities. It was only a small matter for the virus to jump from staff to elderly resident and from elderly resident to other staff and visiting family members and from there onward into the community. My nurse and I had wandered into the heart of the pandemic.

Alarmed, I notified the management of the facility of the need to have infection control procedures, as well as significant retraining of all staff. The response from management was disheartening. No policy for regular staff testing was in place. In fact the director of nursing was unofficially censured for taking the initiative to have patients and staff tested without the approval of the corporate office. Any attempt to convince administration was being met with resistance and foot dragging at every level. With growing concern, I alerted the Chief Medical Officer of HCA Reston Hospital that I had uncovered a viral hot zone and that he should prepare for an influx of very sick individuals.

In two to three weeks, multiple residents had fallen ill, and multiple hospitalizations and deaths had occurred, and the situation was broadcast on the news. The administration finally quarantined infected residents in a sick wing away from healthy residents. I resigned in disgust from that facility, but the situation was unfortunately widespread in all the retirement communities and memory care facilities across the United States. Eldercare is the forgotten underbelly of the US health-care system. Throughout the year 2020, the death rate for age-matched non-nursing home residents was 87 deaths per 100,000 residents. By contrast, the death rate for age-matched nursing home residents was 108-fold higher at about 9,200 per 100,000 residents.[87]

The paper by Cronin and Evans found that the excess mortality among nursing home residents was highly predictable along a quality of nursing home spectrum using CMS five-star ratings of nursing home quality. It is interesting to note that neither high quality (five-star) homes nor one-star homes were able to prevent the entry of COVID disease into their home. But five-star homes were better at containment of spread of disease within the home, using a combination of higher staff-to-resident ratios, earlier case detection, and quicker isolation strategies. In this the saga of the spread of COVID in nursing homes was a mirror of the way the disease spread through US society. Neither could block the entry of the disease into their environment, but the better homes could effectively contain its spread and mitigate its impact through the policies they swiftly implemented. In this the nursing home story was a miniature model, a laboratory of public health policy lessons for all America. Unfortunately, no one was watching or learning.

Across the world, the same story of overcrowding, lack of education, ineptitude, and sheer negligence and malpractice was allowing the disease

---

[87] C. J. Cronin and W. N. Evans, "Nursing Home Quality, COVID-19 Deaths, and Excess Mortality," *J Health Econ* 82 (March 2022): 102,592, doi: 10.1016/j.jhealeco.2022.102592, epub January 21, 2022, PMID: 35104669, PMCID: PMC8776351.

to spread like a forest fire through dry underbrush. In Norway, Sweden and Italy with large retirement and senior communities the death toll was horrific. To us at the frontlines of the conflagration, it felt like we were at war with the devil himself and were witness to the reaper's dance on a vast field of bodies. How this played out across the world and in our homes and businesses had some very common themes. The pandemic brought home in a vivid manner the essential fragility of life and its impermanent nature. We all live with the illusion that we are assured of our next breath and that, after each night, we will wake up the following morning to see the sun. The pandemic blew that illusion apart and brought us face-to-face, eyeball-to-eye socket with the grinning face of death. Confronted by the terror of our own mortality, we saw the fabric of human society ripped apart and the character of people revealed, and the sight was not pretty.

A Need to Predict

My doctor friends play golf in their time off. I train police dogs. I train and compete in a sport called Schutzhund, a German word for "protection dog." I have often said that Schutzhund is a hands-on MBA course in leadership and decision-making. There is nothing that hones your ability to lead as powerfully and as quickly as seeking to control, command, direct, and ultimately partner with another predator species that is gifted with power, agility, and razor-sharp teeth and a crushing bite. It is in training and competing with my German shepherd that I discovered a universal truth about all creatures from an amoeba to a human. This can be summed up in a few aphorisms.

Life is essentially unpredictable. No matter how small or how great a creature may be, life unpredictable in the randomness of its presentation.

All creatures strive to maximize opportunities for pleasurable experiences and minimize the occurrence of unpleasant experiences in their life.

The ability to predict the occurrence of either pleasurable or unpleasant events successfully is the secret to survival because it allows the animal to position itself to secure its advantage in the experience of both. Animals are constantly attempting to figure out what is likely to happen in the next five minutes. A tiger that cannot predict where the deer is likely to appear is going to go hungry. The deer that cannot predict where the tiger will appear is going to get eaten.

Creatures use memory to register patterns of events and circumstances. They use these patterns to predict the probability of what can occur in their immediate future.

This need to predict, born out of the drive for survival, is the basis of learning and behavior.

Finally, leaders who can give reliable cues and guidance that secures predictable outcomes for their teams consistent with the individual and collective desires of the team become sought after and followed.

The pandemic produced intense panic and distress on a global level by making our life and the outcome of our actions unpredictable. In addition to the unpredictability imposed un humans by the virus, the sheer capriciousness, ignorance, and mendacity of the world's leaders in the way they communicated to the public produced chaos in the psyche of the population. This unpredictability was magnified logarithmically in vulnerable populations like the elderly and the cognitively impaired. A person with impaired memory has no way of forming a stable reference point of cues from his environment to guide his choices and actions. In the absence of predictability or even an illusion of predictability, sheer panic sets in. That was the impact of the pandemic in the nursing homes of the world. Overnight, the routines of elderly adults were totally changed, and no one could explain why in a way that would make sense to eighty-five-year-old pops with dementia.

Why can I not walk down this hallway anymore? That is my favorite spot by the window. Why can't I sit there? Where is my daughter (or son)? Why can't I see them anymore? Why are you wearing that thing on your face? Are you coming to my room to rob me? Why is my son standing there outside my window and waving to me? Where is my friend Alice? Where did you take her? I saw those men tie Alice on the rolling bed and take her. Where is she?

The only saving grace is that a lot of the seniors were spared the venom and vitriol that was being spewed in the political rhetoric on the media. But families and seniors suffered the loss of dignity compounded by isolation and loneliness at the end of a life in which, at the very minimum, deserved the familiar caress of a hand and a death faced with the companionship of a loved family member.

CHAPTER 8

Man Who Would Be King

The Prince of Cumberland! That is a step
On which I must fall down, or else o'er leap,
For in my way it lies. Stars, hide your fires;
Let not light see my black and deep desires.
The eye wink at the hand; yet let that be
Which the eye fears, when it is done, to see."

—*Macbeth*

A Fact Sheet

In August 2020, faced with the growing reality of a US death toll in the hundreds of thousands and the rising beat of Democrat campaign drums thundering that the forty-fifth US president and his administration allowed Americans to die rather than risk stock market losses, the Trump White House put out a fact sheet titled "President Trump's Historic Coronavirus Response."[88] In it, the administration set out claims that they had acted with clarity, decisiveness, and leadership that protected Americans; saved lives and businesses; and was effective in its public health response to the pandemic. As a document in an election year

---

[88] https://trumpwhitehouse.archives.gov/briefings-statements/president-trumps-historic-coronavirus-response/

during the greatest global crisis of the century, the Trump document was singular in the extent of its self-serving political rhetoric when compared with facts that were known then and have emerged since.

The key claims of the Trump White House fact sheet were that the Trump administration:

(a) Took early action to cut off travel from China; They did not.

(b) Built the world's leading testing system from nothing; To the contrary the US response struggled with testing for several months after the declaration of the pandemic. Trump himself insisted falsely that increased testing only results in increased number of cases and preferred an ostrich like head in the sand approach to the pandemic. A greater example of wishful denial of reality would be hard to find in the annals of history.

(c) Enacted mitigation measures to slow the spread; The MAGA Republicans flouted masking and lock down measures all through the year 2020.

(d) Mobilized public and private sectors to secure needed supplies; The administration had a late start in this area and did not mobilize effectively until July 2020, 6 months after the first US reported case.

(e) Took action to protect vulnerable Americans; Contrary to this, the opposition to lockdowns and mask mandates by Trump and the MAGA Republicans and the administration's policy of encouraging the spread of infections to accelerate the development of "herd immunity" put elderly and vulnerable Americans at increased risk.

(f) Launched effort to deliver vaccine and therapeutics in record time; This in the form of Operation WARP Speed, was the Trump administrations singular success of the pandemic.

(g) Provided support to workers and businesses; The $2.0 trillion CARES Act of March 2020 was a significant safety net to American workers and businesses.

(h) Paved the way for reopening to get America working again; While America did reopen it is highly doubtful that the administrations action actually paved the way at all. Rather the journey towards reopening was a road filled with ruts, ditches, and potholes that took the life of over 1 million Americans and ruined society, communities and businesses alike.

(i) Surged resources to hot spots as they arose; Far from it, the Trump administration deliberately blocked or delayed the provision of resources to hot spots.

(j) Confronted China as the origin of the virus, while Democrats and the media cowered; In true xenophobic fashion Trump spent much of his time casting xenophobic slurs, calling it the China virus etc. but persisted in spreading false statements about its lethality.

Deadly Lies

On September 15, veteran journalist Bob Woodward of Nixon Watergate fame published his second book on the Trump White House. Woodward's *Rage* covered the Trump administration of 2019 to 2020 and followed his previous book, *Fear*, which chronicled the initial two years of the Trump presidency.[89] In *Rage*, Woodward revealed taped conversations between him and Trump where the president had said as early as February 7 about the SARS-CoV-2 virus, "This is deadly stuff," adding that it was five times as deadly as the flu and acknowledging that the virus was airborne. "That's always tougher than touch. You know, the touch, you don't have to touch things, right? But the air, you just breathe the air, and that's how it's passed."

Yet on February 27, Trump declared that the virus would disappear "like a miracle." He would make statements like, "You have 15 people [with the coronavirus], and the 15 within a couple of days is going to be down to close to zero." But Trump openly admitted to Woodward on

---

[89] Bob Woodward, *Rage* (Simon & Schuster, September 2020).

tape that he played down the lethality of the virus even as he was making these statements and as more American's sickened and cities across the United States were being shut down.

On March 19, Trump admitted, "I wanted to always play it down. I still like playing it down because I don't want to create a panic." While admitting that the virus could affect young as well as elderly people, Trump boasted that his administration had everything under control, insisting on March 24 that the United States would be back to normal by Easter Sunday. "You'll have packed churches all over our country. I think it'll be a beautiful time."

Indeed, on October 2, 2020, the House Select Subcommittee on the Coronavirus Crisis reported that beginning February 2020, the Trump administration was found to have interfered with the coronavirus pandemic response in at least forty-seven documented occasions.[90] The full report which is available online, details actions such as refusal to quarantine infected cruise ship passengers; threats to CDC officials for speaking the truth; differential allocation of resources to democrat leaning states; repeated interference with guidance of the CDC on masking, quarantine and travel advisories; promotion of unproven drugs and medical treatments; interference in procurement and distribution of PPE to the public; ignoring warnings of mass outbreaks in ICE detention centers; interference with the CDC Morbidity and Mortality reports and propagation of misleading projections of death rates;

The list goes on in excruciating detail in a report that is staggering in its scope, detail, and sheer self-serving mendacity.

A Misguided Policy

The overarching theme that runs like a common thread through the various policy decisions and actions of the Trump administration during

---

[90] House oversight committee releases report detailing efforts of Trump administration officials to 'undermine' Covid-19 efforts in US. https://www.cnn.com/2021/12/17/politics/house-committee-trump-covid-19/index.html

the eleven months of 2020 from January 2020 till November 2020 can be summed up in a single sentence.

Do not do anything that can jeopardize reelection!

Every one of the myriads of apparently conflicting and schizophrenic policy switches of the Trump administration during these catastrophic eleven months harmonizes into a uniform pattern when viewed through the transactional lens of this mantra of the constant pursuit and preservation of personal power.

By December 31, 2020, the total number of US cases soared into the stratosphere of excess of 20 million cases. Meanwhile, the Trump administration remained ostrich-like with its head buried in the sand, ruled by a leader who was entrenched in the belief that, if he repeated a lie often enough and with sufficient force, it would become the truth.

Indeed, multiple experts have since concluded that the actions of the Trump administration were directly responsible for up to 40 percent increased number of COVID deaths in the United States and nearly 200,000 excess deaths over what those numbers would have been if the United States had adopted the same policies as its northern neighbor, Canada. [91] In testimony to the US Congress, Dr. Deborah Birx, who led the Trump White House Coronavirus Task Force, bluntly declared that the Trump administration was distracted by the election and neglected to execute an effective pandemic response.

I remember a conversation in the doctors' lounge of my hospital with a colleague of mine who wryly commented on these statistics, saying sarcastically, "When you kill one person you hang for murder. When you kill 200,000, it simply becomes misguided policy."

The incredible irony is that, had Trump responded to the pandemic from day one with a focus on alleviating the toll of human suffering and death instead of trying to save his own reelection, the man who would be king would have become just that.

---

[91] Rebecca Shabad. NBC News Dec 17, 2021. Trump White House made 'deliberate efforts' to undermine Covid response, report says. https://www.nbcnews.com/politics/congress/trump-white-house-made-deliberate-efforts-undermine-covid-response-report-n1286211

CHAPTER 9

The Hope of Heroes

"And will you stay with us," asked Epimetheus, "forever and ever?"

"As long as you need me," said Hope. "And that will be as long as you live in the world. There may be times and seasons when you think I have vanished entirely. But again and again, when perhaps you least expect it, you shall see the glimmer of my wings on the ceiling of your cottage."
—*Hope to Epimetheus, husband of Pandora after the opening of Pandora's box*

Throughout the pandemic, across the world, we were witness to the incredible grace of the human spirit. For all the darkness that was manifested during the pandemic, there was also the simultaneous outpouring of connection and compassion that transcended all geopolitical boundaries and fault lines of color, creed, and beliefs. In the clinic, we were the beneficiaries of spontaneous expressions of love and support from random members of the local community.

Doctors and nurses are human beings too. We are subject to the same foibles of fear, doubt, fatigue, and loss of motivation that plague the rest of humanity. During the pandemic, my staff and I would eat and sleep separated from the rest of our family so we did not bring home to our loved ones the contagion we so freely faced at work. From March

2020 to December 24, 2020, when I received my first shot of the Pfizer vaccine, I would change out of my work clothes in the garage of our house and throw the clothes into the washing machine. I would eat my meal separately from my family, wash the dishes in a separate sink, and sleep in a basement bedroom.

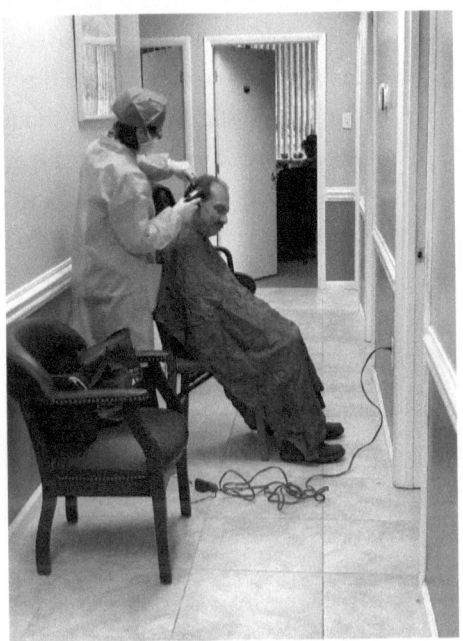

My staff and I even gave each other haircuts in the office so we did not have to go the salon and risk unnecessary exposure. It was a solitary warrior-monk existence of focused abstinence and purpose against an implacable enemy.

All over the world society was waking up to recognize our desperate dependence and need for the everyday heroes of life. Heroes all of them—janitor heroes, postal worker heroes, grocery store worker heroes, farmer and meat packer heroes, health-care heroes. Simple common folk stepped up to reaffirm human connection and fellowship and, by so doing, directly confronted a disease that made all forms of human connection dangerous to human life. The pandemic was humanity's worst of times and best of times. There was no fanfare, no accolades.

These people just showed up and would not back down. While leaders around the world lied and hid, ordinary folks stood up and walked up to the assistance of their fellows, pressing forward against the point of the knife held by the reaper to their throats. They collectively looked death in the eye, and death flinched. A friend of my wife found a large case of hazmat overalls in her office and came over to the clinic and dropped it off, causing my wife to break down in tears of gratitude. I did not realize until then the magnitude of fear my wife was masking behind her stoic support. The owner of the Thai restaurant in the shopping center near my clinic showed up once every week with a large case of fresh Thai food for our staff so we who were deluged with patients and little time to eat would have some sustenance.

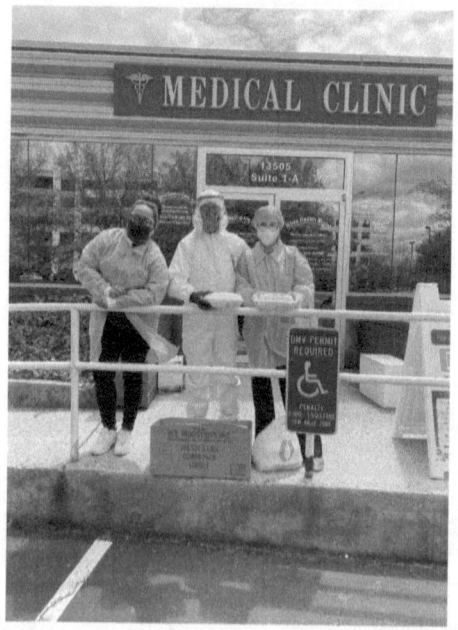

My colleague Dr. Khanna, along with Dr. Chhabra mobilized the membership of the Greater Washington Association of Physicians from India (GWAPI) to conduct a two-pronged drive. For one, GWAPI organized a series of Zoom conferences to teach physicians strategies and best practices to remain open safely and continue to deliver care to their patient populations. At that time, no organization was even thinking about the grassroots physician practices. These lectures with physicians sharing experiences in an each-one-teach-one effort enabled small physician practices to acquire and implement skills that kept them open to deliver incredibly vital health care during a crisis.

In addition, these lectures directly impacted quality of care and education of patient populations in the communities of northern Virginia, suburban Maryland; and the Washington, DC, far more powerfully than any health department communique. The credit for this effort directly goes to Dr. Chhabra and my colleague Dr. Khanna, two of the most practical visionaries in medicine I have known in my forty years as a physician.

But GWAPI did not restrict its efforts to the local communities of the Washington, DC, area. Every day, we physicians were being besieged with desperate calls for help from all over the world. America is a country of immigrants; it is the global melting pot. The physician community of America hails from all over the world, and we were all intimately aware of the crises in the countries of our origin. Whether it was Ukraine, Moldovia, Slovakia, Afghanistan, Vietnam, Bangladesh, Sri Lanka, or India, the physician community in the United States was in constant touch with populations all over the world.

My colleagues and I who were immigrants from India, of course, all had friends and family in India. We were all members of WhatsApp groups of high school networks or medical college networks and were intimately aware of the crisis unfolding in our country of origin. The pandemic had a late start in India. For most of 2020, India was spared the bulk of the impact of the original SARS-CoV-2 virus and its subsequent variants, Alpha, Beta, and Gamma. Prime Minister Modi even bragged at the World Economic Forum's Davos Dialogue on January 28, 2021, that India's proactive public health policies had successfully controlled COVID in the country.[92]

Sixty days later, India was reeling under the impact of the Delta

---

[92] YouTube Video. PM Modi's speech at WEF's Davos summitt. https://www. youtube.com/watch?v=z1h3M4zQXPY&t=251s

variant. Overnight, hospitals were overflowing, and patients were coming by taxies, three-wheeler autos, and private cars in long caravans to health centers, waiting in the oppressive heat of India as they gasped like fish out of water for a breath of life. Oxygen supplies were quickly exhausted all over the country, as oxygen manufacturing plants found demand overwhelming their production capacity even when they were being run 24-7 nonstop. When beds were full, patients were bedded on mattresses beneath beds. There would be one patient on the bed, and beneath the bed, another patient would be lying on a mattress, essentially converting beds into bunk beds. Doctors and nurses would work round the clock with what little they had. When there was no more floor space in the hospital, patients were being treated in the corridors and lawns outside, until eventually the care giving and care receiving would spill over into the parking lot as health-care workers moved between cars and rickshaws to assist with what little they had.

Most of us in the United States are so privileged we cannot conceive of what it means to deliver care in a country like India. It was in this environment that GWAPI launched what was then considered an inconceivable assistance effort. They raised funds for oxygen concentrators, ventilators, autoPAP and BiPAP devices, ICU supplies, masks, and sanitizers. [93] An entrepreneur friend who owned a shipping company, the Punita Group, arranged for containers of these supplies to be shipped to India. On the Indian side, a receiving team of friends of the GWAPI physicians facilitated the customs clearance and security of the shipment to its final destinations to hospitals, health centers, rural clinics all over northern and southern India.

The GWAPI network did not limit themselves to just aid. Key physicians offered themselves as free consultative telemedicine resource to physicians in India. During the day, we would be in the clinic testing

---

[93] Oxygen concentrators are devices the size of portable dehumidifiers that take room air into the oxygen machine, compressing it, purifying it, and removing nitrogen and other impurities and finally delivering the 90 to 95 percent oxygen-enriched air to the patient.

AutoPAP (automatic positive airway pressure) devices blow air and force air into lungs too stiff to expand.

and treating our patients. In the evening, I would go home, and, after dinner, I would go to my basement bedroom, power up my laptop, and begin my second shift of WhatsApp and Zoom video calls to health teams in India. We would discuss X-rays and lab reports and treatment strategies of patients. These conversations would go on till 2:00 a.m. Then I'd switch off and sleep. The next day at 6:30 a.m. would be a new day, and the grind would begin again.

When I look back at these past three years, there is a sense of deep satisfaction and pride over what we individually and collectively accomplished. There, too, is an immense feeling of blessedness over what I can only call the hand of Providence that has sheltered my team, my colleagues, and myself. Indeed, to think we were able to waltz cheek to jowl with the reaper a mere six to nine inches from patients' faces as they coughed and sneezed on us while we were testing them with only a curtain of fabric and plastic separating us is mind-blowing. The struggle, the fatigue, the isolation of those times pales into insignificance before the magnitude of what was achieved globally by hundreds of thousands of ordinary people. The virus may have spread like a cloud across the globe, but it was neutralized by the committed will of hundreds of thousands of individuals who networked and proved that the essence of what it means to be human was alive and well.

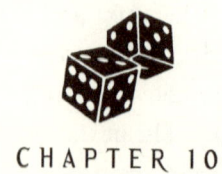

CHAPTER 10

Vaccines and Violence

Barn's burnt down — Now I can see the moon.
—Mizuta Masahide

Warp Speed

The COVID-19 pandemic is a story of broken records. Just as the United States was never inepter in its public health management as during this pandemic, so also never in the history of humankind has an effective vaccine been created from concept to finished product in eight months instead of the usual eight to ten years. In this, at least some credit must be accorded to the Operation Warp Speed of the Trump administration. By early April 2020, globally, an astonishing 110 potential different COVID-19 vaccines were in development. For all the urgency of the pandemic, none of the vaccine development efforts were at that time envisaging a timeline of development to delivery of less than two years. By contrast, Operation Warp Speed was an American governmental effort to put the full, unrestricted weight of all the resources wielded by the US government; scientific, academic, and diverse governmental agencies; the military; and the private sector in a concerted effort to create 300 million doses of an effective vaccine by October-November 2020 reserved entirely for administration into American arms.[94]

If there was one man who can be singled out, who stood behind this effort, it would be Moncef Slaoui. Few individuals could have had more diversity of background and character than Slaoui. An immunologist by training, he hailed from Morocco and was the former head of vaccines at Glaxo Smith-Kline with a history of revolutionary militant radicalism as a student and a registered Democrat in a rabidly Republican administration.[95] Yet Slaoui is unreserved in his praise for President Trump regarding Operation Warp Speed. In a statement to Science on January 25, 2021, Slaoui is emphatically direct regarding Trump, stating that though he completely disagrees with his (Trump's) values and qualities he projects as a leader, he felt that Warp Speed was a visionary alignment of public and private sector resources. [96]

Slaoui who insists that both Trump and Jared Kushner never interfered with his ability to execute, speaks of Warp Speed with pride and affection for the entire effort and the team that accomplished it, as well as with some sadness at what he sees as unfortunate politicization of the success of that effort. Together with General Gustav Perna, co-leader of Operation Warp Speed with Slaoui, the Warp Speed duo marshalled an incredible team of cross-disciplinary capabilities in a revolutionary public-private sector partnership to move five vaccines from concept to Phase III clinical trials of which two were fully authorized for administration in eight months (May 2020 to December 2020).

---

[94] Jon Cohen. Science May 12, 2020. Unveiling 'Warp Speed', the White House's America-first push for a coronavirus vaccine. https://www.science.org/content/article/unveiling-warp-speed-white-house-s-america-first-push-coronavirus-vaccine

[95] As a student in Belgium, Slaoui was part of a secret militant organization that wanted to spark a revolution in Morocco.

[96] Jon Cohen. Science. Jan 25, 2021. Proud of vaccine success, Warp speed's ex-science head talks, politics, presidents, and future pandemics. https://www.science.org/content/article/proud-vaccine-success-warp-speed-s-ex-science-head-talks-politics-presidents-and-future

Designer Vaccines to Cancer Drugs

The story of the mRNA vaccine is a story of four decades of solitary, passionate struggle on the part of one lone scientist at the University of Pennsylvania that eventually blossomed into a breakthrough technology. That breakthrough resulted in a miracle drug that saved millions. It now holds the promise of the creation of vaccines for other notoriously resistant infectious diseases, such as malaria, tuberculosis, and leprosy, and of ending cancer, that ancient scourge of humankind. On a personal level, I have, in decades past in India, worked with teams dedicated to creating a vaccine for leprosy and tuberculosis as part of my doctoral work. I first met my wife at the National Institute of Immunology and All India Institute of Medical Sciences, New Delhi, India, during a collaboration between my lab and hers on creating immune-reactive peptide fragments for generation of a malaria vaccine.

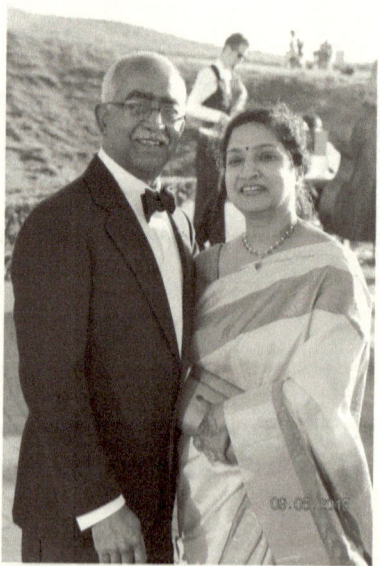

PC: Dr. Madhav Swaminathan, MD

So, the story of the mRNA vaccine and the promise of this technology resonates at a fundamental level with my psyche. It is important to understand that a vaccine is simply a method of teaching the body's immune system to first recognize a foreign molecular structure and then to bind and destroy that structure. Think of our body's immune system as a powerful multifunctional law enforcement agency. The process of immune recognition is like biometric printing and recognition of a felon in a vast law enforcement database that is accessible in an instant. The next time a microbe with the same biometrics enters the body, it is recognized and neutralized right at the point of entry. When this is accomplished successfully, the body very effectively blocks any infectious agent—viral, bacterial, protozoal, or parasitic—from gaining a foothold in the body and destroys the agent then and there.

A powerful immunity is the very best mask protection that one can ever conceive of—the very best protection against any attack. The body can learn this defense in two ways, (1) by prior exposure to the infectious agent during actually contracting the disease and recovering from it and (2) by receiving a vaccine. So, while surviving a natural infection is nature's method of vaccinating us, it is, of course, fraught with the risk of residual damage and even death. Vaccination gives the body's immune system an opportunity to learn to recognize and neutralize the pathogen without running the risk of contracting the full-blown disease itself and all the attendant ills.

The first vaccines ever developed used either heat-inactivated pathogens or live pathogens that were attenuated ("weakened") in some way, such that they were unable to cause disease but were able to serve as suitable targets of recognition to teach the immune system how to recognize them. An alternate method was using a close relative of the actual pathogen that would not cause serious disease in humans but was sufficiently similar in structure to serve as an immune system recognition target. Thus, in 1796, the British doctor Edward Jenner used pustular material from a patient of cowpox to inoculate a young boy who subsequently became immune to smallpox.

From that point on, for the next two centuries, there has been an explosion of knowledge in the fields of microbiology, virology, immunology, and vaccinology. However, the strategies have remained nearly the same; use (1) live attenuated organisms, (2) inactivated organisms or fragments thereof, or (3) closely related but less pathogenic species as immunological targets for the development of immune recognition and immunity.

Powerful as this method has been and though it has been credited with the eradication of many lethal infectious scourges of humankind, there are significant limitations. There are a sizeable number of organisms that evade immune recognition by hiding themselves from the immune system. Some of them do this by residing inside human cells and wreaking their mischief within. Thus, the malarial parasite, Lyme disease, leishmaniasis, the microbe of syphilis and sleeping sickness are some intracellular pathogens that, to this day, continue to cause havoc in many areas of the world. Others evade recognition by presenting nonessential portions of themselves to the immune system, thus fooling the immune system into creating antibodies that are useless for the purpose of destroying the pathogen. Still other pathogens have molecular structures that actively interfere with the immune cell communication networks that coordinate the process of immune recognition and antibody generation.

In the case of COVID-19, there are seven such escape strategies for the SARS-CoV-2 virus:[97]

1. Camouflage of the spike proteins by sugar molecules to evade recognition
2. Direct interference of the mechanisms by which portions of viral proteins are cut up by the human system and presented to the immune system by a sophisticated molecular immune recognition system called MHC-I antigen presentation.
3. Inhibition of synthesis of a human immune cytokine called interferon that teaches immune cells to attack the virus
4. Viral interference of a human cellular defense mechanism called "apoptosis" that would result in viral infected cells committing

[97] A. Rubio-Casillas, E. M. Redwan, and V. N. Uversky, "SARS-CoV-2: A Master of Immune Evasion," *Biomedicines* 10, no. 6 (June 7, 2022): 1,339.

accelerated death, a kind of cellular suicide, rather than serve as viral replication factories.

5. Direct cell-to-cell infection promoted by viral infected human cells to directly connect with neighboring cells through cellular nanotubes to directly transmit infective virus to adjacent cells through these channels and, thereby, evade exposure to the immune system cells lurking outside.

6. Direct cell-to-cell infection by web formation of connections (syncytia formation) between virus-infected and uninfected cells

7. Release of infective virus from infected human cells in cellular blebs called exosomes that fuse with neighboring uninfected cells, thereby bypassing the ACE2 receptor mediated attachment and entry mechanism and allowing for infection into human cells and tissue that may not express the ACE2 receptor on their surface

These escape mechanisms of the virus are the primary reason why using inactivated SARS-CoV-2 virus as a vaccine (as done by the Chinese Sinovax) results in a less potent vaccine than other versions.

These and other problems in achieving immune recognition to complex molecular targets have, for decades, enticed scientists to come up with the development of synthetic molecular targets for the immune system's recognition. With the advent of molecular biology and genetic technology, scientists had the ability to synthesize fragments of an organism's protein structure in the lab and then use these fragments as vaccines. The problems now were selecting the right targets and administering them in the right mixture of adjuvants for triggering a successful immunological response. But it soon became apparent that mere fragments of microbial proteins (called peptides) were not sufficient. In real life, these proteins were covered in sugar residues through a process called glycosylation such that the actual immunological target in real life was the peptide-sugar molecule. So, unless scientists could devise a way of synthetically duplicating the glycosylation process, it would not work. Enter the concept of mRNA technology.

The story of Katalin Karikó is one of an immigrant genius struggling within a hostile establishment of stereotypical barriers and discrimination and sustained by little else than a bright, burning flame of belief in a vision of the possible. A Hungarian biochemist, Dr. Karikó had an academic excellence that manifested early. In her native Hungary as an eighth grader, Karikó won the third prize in a national biology contest. As early as 1978, she was working to develop a methodology for delivering short RNA molecules into cells as a step in the creation of RNA-driven antiviral therapeutics. It would be more than four decades before her dream would materialize into reality.

Dr. Karikó emigrated to the United States in 1985, originally as a postdoctoral fellow in the lab of Robert Suhadolnik at Temple University to continue her work in RNA therapeutics. She moved to the University of Pennsylvania in 1989 as a nontenure track research assistant professor and began her work on mRNA therapeutics. What followed was sixteen lonely years of failure and rejection. Karikó's idea was essentially simple: (1) Synthesize the mRNA that codes for a specific biologically active protein. (2) Inject the mRNA into cells, sit back, and watch the cells read the mRNA and synthesize the protein encoded by it. (3) Measure the biological effect that the synthesized protein exerts within the cell. In theory, using such a method, you could deliver the instructions to a cell to literally synthesize its own drug within it. A whole field of targeted therapeutics would open.

Karikó's ideas were rejected as too "pie-in-the-sky"—idle fantasies of a crazy Hungarian woman scientist. When injected, mRNA would trigger a severe allergic reaction that would kill the mice, rendering the experiment a bust even before it could start. Experiment after experiment failed. The months became years, and the failures and the ridicule mounted.

But the constant and stinging academic ridicule at the University of Pennsylvania met its match in the strong support of fellow scientists Drew Weissman, Elliot Barnathan, and David Langer, whose faith in and encouragement of her ideas was persistent. A breakthrough came in 2004, when Karikó noticed that transfer RNA (tRNA), a form of

RNA in the cell, does not trigger the same lethal allergic reaction that mRNA did. The difference between the two was that tRNA contained a modified nucleoside called pseudo-uridine, whereas mRNA contained uridine. Karikó created a new batch of mRNA, substituting pseudo-uridine in place of uridine, and the mice survived!

The paper describing this in 2005 was rejected by Nature within twenty-four hours of submission as not innovative and was published in Immunity.[98] A subsequent paper in 2008 expanded on the superior properties of nucleoside-substituted mRNAs.[99] But institutional recognition at UPenn continued to evade Karikó.

Finally in 2013, at the age of fifty-eight, Dr. Karikó left UPenn to join a small pharmaceutical company, BioNtech to continue her mRNA work. In 2017, Dr. Karikó, together with several scientists from multiple institutions, including Drew Weissman, were able to show that a single fifty-microgram dose of nucleoside-modified mRNA vaccine was able to protect monkeys from Zika virus.[100] The field of mRNA vaccine technology had begun.

Right at the outset, it became obvious to everyone that mRNA technologies greatest strength was the speed of manufacture possible

---

[98] K. Karikó, M. Buckstein, H. Ni, and D. Weissman, "Suppression of RNA Recognition by Toll-like Receptors: The Impact of Nucleoside Modification and the Evolutionary Origin of RNA," *Immunity* 23 (2005), 165–75.

[99] K. Karikó, H. Muramatsu, F. A. Welsh, J. Ludwig, H. Kato, S. Akira, and D. Weissman, "Incorporation of Pseudouridine into mRNA Yields Superior Nonimmunogenic Vector with Increased Translational Capacity and Biological Stability," *Mol Ther* 16, no. 11 (November 2008): 1,833–40, doi: 10.1038/mt.2008.200, epub September 16, 2008, PMID: 18797453; PMCID: PMC2775451.

[100] N. Pardi, M. J. Hogan, R. S. Pelc, H. Muramatsu, H. Andersen, C. R. DeMaso, K. A. Dowd, L. L. Sutherland, R. M. Scearce, R. Parks, W. Wagner, A. Granados, J. Greenhouse, M. Walker, E. Willis, J. S. Yu, C. E. McGee, G. D. Sempowski, B. L. Mui, Y. K. Tam, Y. J. Huang, D. Vanlandingham, V. M. Holmes, H. Balachandran, S. Sahu, M. Lifton, S. Higgs, S. E. Hensley, T. D. Madden, M. J. Hope, K. Karikó, S. Santra, B. S. Graham, M. G. Lewis, T. C. Pierson, B. F. Haynes, and D. Weissman, "Zika Virus Protection by a Single Low-Dose Nucleoside-Modified mRNA Vaccination," *Nature* 543, no. 7,644 (March 9, 2017): 248–251, doi: 10.1038/nature21428, epub February, 2017, PMID: 28151488, PMCID: PMC5344708.

and the vast ability to scale up production. Karikó described its principal advantage as speed of manufacture. Using her method, a scientist can order and receive a gene of interest in 1 to 2 days and use it as a template to make mRNA in a few hours. The mRNA can be transfected into cells to produce a significant amount of target protein for use in an additional few hours and the costs involved are relatively trivial considering the scale. The entire process is immensely scaleable which lends to its attractiveness from a commercial perspective since everything can be done in a single pot.[101]

Dr. Katalin Karikó's lonely forty-one-year journey through the wilderness of scientific opinion was over. She would emerge as the prophet who would save humankind.

Last-Mile Stumble

In April 2020, when Moncef Slaoui took on Operation Warp Speed, he knew it would be mRNA technology he would have to place his bets on. Nothing else would produce an effective vaccine fast enough to save humanity. But the success of Warp Speed was marred by missteps in the administration of the vaccine, the final mile of the entire immunization effort. In this, Slaoui puts the blame squarely at the weakness and fragmentation of America's public health network at the state level, which was responsible for the actual distribution to the population.

Slaoui could not be more accurate in his analysis. As a physician in the trenches, I can personally attest to the immense difficulty I had in procuring vaccine doses for administration to my patient population when the first doses were made available on December 12, 2020. When the first doses of Pfizer and Moderna mRNA vaccines were made available, the policy was to first vaccinate the vaccinators—to immunize America's health-care workforce, who could then turn around and immunize the population of their communities. In addition, these

---

[101] Prashant Nair. Proc. Natl. Acad. Sci. Dec 13, 2021. QnAs with Katalin Kariko. https://www.pnas.org/doi/10.1073/pnas.2119757118

vaccines required complex storage conditions at -80° Centigrade, with a limited shelf life of a maximum of thirty days at temperatures higher than that. So, the initial vaccination centers became major hospital centers and regional health department clinics.

This by itself was a good first step—or it would have been if it had not remained at that level for another six months. I received my own dose of Pfizer vaccine on December 24, 2020, at Inova Fairfax Hospital Center, Falls Church, Virginia. My wife as immediate family of a health care worker received hers a few weeks later at the Regional Health Department vaccination center. But then when I tried to procure doses for administration to my patients at my clinic, I was repeatedly rebuffed. It was not until May 2021 that vaccine doses were made available to community physicians and clinics for community administration.

In this debacle, the fault can be squarely placed on two entities—the local health apparatus at the state level and the Trump administration. Even though the vaccine rollout took place in the Biden administration, the process and roadblocks and, most importantly, the inertia generated by the mentality of the Trump administration took six months to reverse and put in place a new method of doing things. The United States of America is a juggernaut, a huge ocean liner, and it cannot turn on a dime just for the wishing of it. It needs time to implement complex supply and distribution channels. And the previous administration had allowed a lot of these capabilities to decay during its four years of grift and self-preservation.

Scorched Earth

Donald Trump realized in late October 2020 that neither Pfizer nor Moderna would have data on the efficacy of their vaccines available before the November 3 elections. This meant there would be no vaccine approved by the FDA before the elections. Trump's paranoia led him to believe this was a conspiracy against him, though Slaoui explained this is not how such matters work. Regardless, Trump essentially washed his hands of the entire effort from that point. He declared the federal government's responsibility was limited to making the vaccine available. Distribution would be up to the diverse state health authorities. As far as he was concerned, in his transactional world view, Warp Speed would not help his reelection, so he could not be concerned about its success.

In fact, in the months between November 2020 and January 2021, the Trump administration actively resisted coordination and transfer of information about Warp Speed and other pandemic-related public health efforts to the incoming Biden administration. In a perverse manner typical of the administration's schizophrenic leadership pattern, failure of the vaccine effort was now of greater political value to the outgoing Republican leadership as much as its success was of value to the Biden administration. In this, the continued illness and death toll of the suffering American populace was of no concern. It was a cynical scorched earth policy of a vindictive, despotically bankrupt regime in desperate retreat.

Given that distribution was the problem of the states, it followed that vaccine distribution was heavily influenced by the political leaning at the state level. The virulent anti-masking rhetoric propagated pre-December 2020 by the Republican leadership evolved into vaccine resistance and anti-vaxxer rhetoric post December 2020. Conspiracy theories flourished. Vaccines, they claimed, contained nano chips that can track people. Vaccines contained magnetic particles detectable by secret government scanners in a vast conspiracy to track the movement of populations. Vaccines would modify the genetic material of people and so on and so forth. These myths were resistant to debunking precisely because they satisfied an underlying belief that has been the basis of much of Republican America's deepest fear—the loss of their own power over their destiny in an America steadily becoming less white; browner and blacker; and more diverse ethnically, culturally, sexually, and economically.

The Venom of Vaccine Misinformation

In my clinic, we were finally approved as a COVID vaccination center in May 2021 and were able to offer both Pfizer and Moderna mRNA vaccine to all comers on a walk-in basis with no prior appointment required. Still, I had to face anti-vaxxer misinformation and vaccine hesitancy on a nearly daily basis. The following is a typical conversation that ended well (though not every conversation had a happy outcome):

Sarah. Doc! I don't know if I want to get the vaccine. I've heard so many rumors about it being unsafe and causing more harm than good.

Me. Sarah, those rumors are just that—rumors. The vaccines have been thoroughly tested and have been proven to be safe and effective in preventing COVID-19. With the help of vaccination, you can save yourself and your loved ones from a serious illness.

Sarah. But what about all the reports of people getting sick after getting the vaccine? I don't want to take that kind of risk.

Me. Much of that is overstated. Yes, you will have some injection site soreness for three days or so, and you will have some flu-like aches, pains, and feverishness in the first twenty-four hours. But that is proof the vaccine is working and your immune system is responding and learning to recognize, fight, and destroy the virus.

The fact is, getting COVID-19 is much more dangerous and can lead to serious health problems, hospitalization, and even death. The vaccines have been shown to greatly reduce the risk of getting sick from COVID-19.

Sarah. Is this really true?

Me. When you examine the record of vaccination, any negative effects that individuals experienced happened within two months. People now have been using these immunizations for more than six months across the globe. Millions have been vaccinated, and they are doing fine. Researchers have observed nothing, and the conclusion is that vaccination has saved a lot of lives.

Most of my patients would understand my arguments and the data I presented and realize they wanted to do their part in protecting themselves and their community from the virus. They would get vaccinated and encourage others to do the same.

As more and more people in the town got vaccinated, the rumors about the vaccine being unsafe started to dissipate. People saw the positive impact that vaccination was having on their health and their community, and they realized the importance of getting vaccinated.

But unfortunately, not every one of my patients fell in that category. One such story is of a very good friend of mine, who I shall call Bill. Bill ran a very successful auto repair shop and is one of the best vehicle maintenance and body shop persons in my area. A man of twenty-four-karat integrity, Bill is who I've always trusted with all my automotive problems. His wife and family lived in a farm out in the horse country surrounded by Virginian vineyards and were simply the best kind of people you could find on earth.

Yet for all this, Bill would not get vaccinated. He was too polite to say no to my face, but he'd keep changing the topic every time I tried to get him to do it. I recognized his hesitancy, and I respected him too much to push my views down his throat. So, I let it ride and prayed inwardly he would escape a visit from the reaper. But that was not to be.

One day, Anne called me in a panic. She was out of town, and Bill was back home alone on the farm. He was running a fever of 104° Fahrenheit. This was when all we had was the vaccine. Paxlovid was not yet available. I called Bill, but no answer. I called Anne back. She had gotten through to Bill in the meanwhile. I gave Anne instructions to make sure Bill had plenty of fluids and rest. She would be home the next morning.

The next morning, I called Anne. She was home, but she was scared. Bill was not looking good. She'd never seen him like this before. He was not fully coherent, speaking sense sometimes and lapsing into nonsense at other times.

I packed my mobile COVID kit and drove the thirty miles to the farm. Gowning up on the lawn outside their house, I walked into the log cabin home Bill had built. Bill was weak and could barely sit straight as I drew some blood and checked his vitals and his oxygenation. He was dehydrated.

I called the local hospital. They were full, but I spoke to the director of the ER who I knew from when I had been the department chair. He found Bill a room.

In six hours, Bill got IV fluids, anti-COVID monoclonal antibodies and Remdesivir, and some steroids. The hospital physician later told me Bill was lucky and had narrowly escaped landing in the ICU on a vent.

Two weeks later, Bill would tell me that night alone on the farm, with Anne being away was the scariest time of his life. He insisted he could feel the virus invading and multiplying in his brain, and it drove him crazy. He said, "Ravi, you have no idea how intensely I prayed that night. I had these crazy thoughts driving me insane, telling me to take my gun and end it right then and there. I prayed to God like I have never done before, not because I feared death or disease. That night I felt I was standing at the edge of the abyss and looking down into hell. A thousand voices were screaming, 'Jump,' and I did not want to go there."

Three months later, Bill walked into my office and received his Pfizer vaccine. His wife, Anne, did not get vaccinated. I have never asked her why. And to this date, I do not know if she ever did.

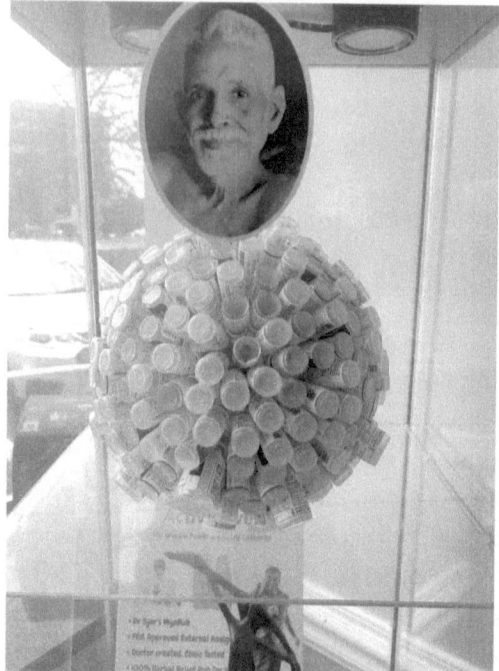

SARS-CoV-2 virus model created out of spent Pfizer and Moderna vaccine vials by student interns at the Iyer Clinic

Stop the Steal

Despite all his support of Operation Warp Speed, at no point has President Trump come out in active, aggressive defense of vaccines and promotion of vaccination. Even when the First Family received their own vaccinations in December, it was done quietly without fanfare or announcement, and Trump never once made a public exhortation that people should follow his example and get themselves vaccinated. At a moral level alone, the spectacle of a leader quietly taking steps to protect himself and his family from a deadly disease without attempting to influence the people he leads to do the same is reprehensible by any standard of humanity. In this, President Trump, the Republican party, and the conservative media is bound to be judged severely by the weight of history.

The anti-vaxxer propaganda also dovetailed as the subtext of the larger Stop the Steal campaign of the postelection Trump strategy. From November 3, 2020, to the date of this writing in spring 2023, Trump has propagated the narrative that the election was stolen from him. In what has since been widely dismissed as the "Great Lie," Trump and, initially, much of the Republican political apparatus actively worked to propagate the narrative that rampant fraud and manipulation was the basis of Trump's dramatic loss on November 3, 2020. This Stop the Steal rhetoric merged with the anti-vaxxer rhetoric and QAnon conspiracy theories to create a vast misinformation conversation that grew and fed the militant fantasies of the alt-right.

On January 6, 2021, the poison of this misinformation spilled over on the streets of Washington, DC, as the infamous insurrection and riot on Capitol Hill to halt Congress from certifying the results of the 2020 presidential elections. Always the master puppeteer, Trump remained in the White House, after exhorting the crowd of Oath Keepers, Proud Boys, and others to fight for their rights by marching on the US Capitol. He watched the violence erupt from the safety of his television room. The murderous melee would eventually end in the death of some rioters and several Capitol Hill police officers and threaten the lives of all the senators and the vice president assembled within the US Congress in the only seditious insurrection the United States of America has ever known.

CHAPTER 11

Virulence and Variants

Two aspects of a virus in action: transmissibility and virulence.

—David Quammen

Every emerging virus that infects the human species for the very first time displays high virulence and pathogenicity because the virus is entering a virgin species with no innate immunity against it. From that point onward, evolution takes over. Each person who is infected generates a billion copies of the virus. This replication of the viral genome is accomplished by the human cell's gene replication machinery.

In normal human genome replication, gene-editing and error-correcting mechanisms are working simultaneously as the human chromosome is copied, ensuring the copy of each chromosome is a faithful replica of the parent chromosome. But this error-correcting mechanism is not as perfect when the human replication machinery is being recruited to read and copy viral genetic material. Therefore, random errors creep in as the viral genetic material is copied and new virions are being packaged. Each of these errors is, in essence, a mutation. That virion containing the mutation is essentially a variant.

Each SARS-CoV-2-infected human cell in a patient is generating a billion new virions. If these random errors were to occur even once every million copies, then there would be a thousand variants emerging from that single cell. A single patient may have trillions of cells infected with the virus. Now you can see how quickly the math adds up. So, the prime fact that should be remembered is that every infected patient is essentially a variant-creating machine.

This is the real reason people should mask up, should isolate, should socially distance, and should vaccinate. They should take these steps so that, if they are infected, they do not spread the variants they create into other people. If they are not infected, they will not receive the variants being released by other infected people.

Now, it is not like the virus has an intelligence that is plotting the creation of variants. This is simply occurring as a mechanical consequence of the virus-copying process. It is stochastic—mere mathematical chance. The process is sloppy, and therefore, variants are created.

Now, most of the variants die out because the underlying error results in a virion that does not infect other people as well as the parent virus. But like a roll of dice on a craps table, if you have unlimited money and time and roll the dice enough, eventually you, too, will win. The virus needs to win only once in billions of copies, and when that happens, a variant has been created that is able to transmit better to the next patient or causes more severe disease. Thus, the original wild-type SARS-CoV-2 virus that prevailed from November 2019 to March 2020 got replaced by the Alpha variant and then successively by the Beta variant. the Gamma variant, the Delta variant and, finally, now the Omicron variant.

Now comes a curious dilemma. In nature, the most successful viruses, from the standpoint of causing disease, are not the most lethal viruses. Rather, they are the most transmissible. A virus that kills its host very quickly will die out faster than it can spread. Similarly, if a virus is highly pathogenic —that is, it causes intense disease very quickly after infection—then that virus also will not spread widely; it will become obvious to others that the infected person is diseased, and they will naturally stay away from the infected person. Such a virus will have a reduced opportunity to spread.

While the actual relationship between transmissibility, pathogenicity, and immune escape is more complex, the ideal candidate for a pandemic would be a virus that is airborne, transmits very well, and causes delayed onset of disease but continues to be dispersed in respiration even before the disease is visible.[102] SARS-CoV-2 was a dream virus created for a pandemic.

Still, the original virus had one flaw. It was lethal. That is bad news for a virus with dreams of global domination. But never mind, nature had trillions of opportunities to get its act together and refine its creation. Analysis of the Alpha, Beta, Gamma, Delta, and Omicron variants revealed a clear progression of better and better fitness for the purpose finding that sweet spot between transmissibility and virulence.[103] Each variant had mutations in the structure of the spike protein that rendered the virus more able to (a) undergo activation of the spike protein by cleavage of the S1 subunit from the S2 subunit, (b) undergo more efficient virion packaging, and (c) undergo immunological escape. This is what evolution is all about. Right before our eyes, over the past two and a half years, the SARS-CoV-2 virus has been evolving to develop greater and greater fitness for its own existence as a viral infection of humans.

This is the natural evolution of every virus that jumps from the animal kingdom to the human species. Initially, it will be highly lethal and significantly transmissible, but it will steadily evolve into variant strains that will transmit better and better and be progressively less lethal to its host. Indeed, this is precisely what the authors of the paper in Nature argue.

Much of the analysis of variants has focused on mutations in the

---

[102] Gkikas Magiorkinis, "On the Evolution of SARS-CoV2 and the Emergence of Variants of Concern," *Trends in Microbiology* (January 2023), https://www.cell.com/trends/microbiology/fulltext/S0966-842X(22)00291-8.

[103] Christiaan van Dorp, Emma Goldberg, Ruian Ke, Nick Hengartner, and Ethan Romero-Severson, "Global Estimates of the Fitness Advantage of SARS-CoV-2 Variant Omicron," *Virus Evolution* 8, no. 2 (2022): veac089, https://doi.org/10.1093/ve/veac089; Roberto Burioni, "Has SARS-COV-2 Reached Peak Fitness?" *Nature Medicine* 27 (2021): 1,323–24, https://www.nature.com/articles/s41591-021-01421-7.

structure of the spike protein. Proteins are formed of a string of amino acids. Each amino acid has a specific shape and configuration and electrical charge, and they interact with their neighboring amino acids to bend, twist, and fold the long string into a specific shape that gives the protein its unique form. Form precedes fitness for function. The spike protein of SARS-CoV-2 has the shape and the function it does because of its specific amino acids and the order in which they occur in the chain. The sequence of amino acids in a protein is called its primary structure, and this is determined by the genetic code for that protein. So, when an error during replication causes a mutation in the genetic code of the virus and when this mutation happens to fall within the portion of the viral genome encoding the spike protein, then the structure of the spike protein changes.

Some structural changes result in no change in function. Some changes result in a reduction in function. Some changes result in enhancement of function. It is simply a random roll of the reaper's dice, and every now and then, it comes up snake eyes.

Thus, a mutation wherein a single nucleotide in position 23,405 in the viral genome of the original Wuhan SARS-CoV-2 strain was changed from adenosine to a guanosine resulted in the infamous D614G change in the sequence of the spike protein amino acid chain.[104] In this, the 614th amino acid in the spike protein was changed from aspartic acid to glycine. This single amino acid change resulted in an increase in the spike protein's ability to bind to its target, the human ACE2 receptor. The D614G mutation is found in every variant from that point onward and has become conserved through the subsequent evolution of the virus through the Alpha, Beta, Gamma, Kappa, and now the Omicron

---

[104] B. Korber, W. M. Fischer, S. Gnanakaran, H. Yoon, J. Theiler, W. Abfalterer, N. Hengartner, E. E. Giorgi, T. Bhattacharya, B. Foley, K. M. Hastie, M. D. Parker, D. G. Partridge, C. M. Evans, T. M. Freeman, and T. I. de Silva, Sheffield COVID-19 Genomics Group, C. McDanal, L. G. Perez, H. Tang, A. Moon-Walker, S. P. Whelan, C. C. LaBranche, E. O. Saphire, and D. C. Montefiori, "Tracking Changes in SARS-CoV-2 Spike: Evidence that D614G Increases Infectivity of the COVID-19 Virus," *Cell* 182, no. 4 (August 20, 2020): 812–27, e19, doi: 10.1016/j.cell.2020.06.043, epub July 3, 2020, PMID: 32697968, PMCID: PMC7332439.

variants and their subvariants, indicating its importance in conferring an enhanced fitness for transmission and infection on the virus.

Another well-known mutation is the E484K mutation, or the "EEK mutant."[105] The negatively charged amino acid glutamic acid in position 484 on the spike protein is replaced with the positively charged amino acid lysine. The EEK mutation is an escape mutation because it confers immune escape properties on the virus. Variants carrying the EEK mutation are not well recognized by monoclonal antibodies directed against the spike protein, thereby thwarting the protection conferred by the immune system. This mutation impacts vaccine efficacy. Some mutations confer both immune escape, as well as enhanced ACE2 receptor binding upon the virus, for example the L452R (leucine 452 to arginine).[106]

The various mutations and the variants that arise from them are classified in a formal lineage called PANGOLIN (Phylogenetic Assignment of Named Global Outbreak Lineages). The mutations that occur in SARS-CoV-2 virus variants are not stories of continuous progression. It is not as if a variant will acquire a mutation like D614G, and then subsequent variants will all carry that mutation and acquire additional new ones. Instead, it is a fascinatingly morbid tale of mutations that emerge and then disappear as new mutations emerge that make old mutations meaningless for the viruses' spread.

For example, the D614G mutation has been preserved through Alpha, Beta, Gamma, Delta, and Omicron variants. But some mutations like the P681 are interesting. The 681 position is the furin cleavage site that is required for separation of the S1 and S2 units of the spike protein.[107] Initially in the Alpha variant, the amino acid proline at this position was changed to the basic amino acid histidine (P681H), making this cleavage site more easily cleavable. Then this mutation disappeared

[105] Jacqui Wise. *BMJ* 2021;372:n359 Covid-19: The E484K mutation and the risks it poses. https://www.bmj.com/content/372/bmj.n359
[106] Zhang, Y., Zhang, T., Fang, Y. *et al.* SARS-CoV-2 spike L452R mutation increases Omicron variant fusogenicity and infectivity as well as host glycolysis. *Sig Transduct Target Ther* 7, 76 (2022). https://www.nature.com/articles/s41392-022-00941-z
[107] Described in chapter 4 "The Face of the Reaper: The Spike"

in the Beta and Gamma variants, only to reappear in the Delta variant. But this time, instead of P681H, the Delta variant had P681R, where the proline amino acid was changed to arginine, which is even more basic than histidine, resulting in a huge boost in S1/S2 cleavage and an increase in transmissibility and infectivity. Then in the Omicron variant, this mutation reverted to the P681H model.

By contrast, the E484K (EEK) mutation that confers immune escape appeared first in the Beta and Gamma variants and then disappeared in the Delta variant, only to reappear in the Omicron variant but this time as the E484A (glutamic acid to alanine) change. The L452R mutation that confers both enhanced receptor binding and enhanced immune escape appeared in the Delta variant and then disappeared in the first strain of the Omicron variant, only to reappear in the latest Omicron strains BA.4, BA.5, and the BQ1.1

Each variant, therefore, may be best described as a new car model. The base chassis is the same, but new models with better and more desirable features (mutations) are being constantly created, and old ones, retired or brought back as the virus continues to evolve toward a best fitness in its place with relation to its human host. It is a burglar constantly refining its housebreaking, entering, and plundering tools.

This is why moving forward beyond 2023, SARS-CoV-2 will now exist as an endemic seasonal infection much like the flu. It is for this reason that we will most probably need annual immunizations against SARS-CoV-2 like we do for the flu. It is to our advantage to keep pushing the vaccine immunity envelope with better and "fitter" vaccines in this arms race between us and the virus.

In addition, there is a small probability that a phenomenon called super-immunity may result in long-lasting immunity against SARS-CoV-2. It is now recognized that there are a small percentage of individuals who develop a robust immunity to SARS-CoV-2, as well as other coronaviruses that render them super-immune to all coronaviruses. It is becoming apparent that these fortunate few have, in addition to antibodies, a high titer of killer T-cells that destroy the virus at the port of entry.[108] Initial studies strongly suggest that the development of this super-immunity requires recognition and immune targeting of viral proteins other than the spike protein of the virus.[109] It now remains for scientists to find a way to reproduce the conditions where this will reliably happen in all immunized individuals.

---

[108] P. Moss, "The T Cell Immune Response against SARS-CoV-2," *Nat Immunol* 23 (2022): 186–93, https://doi.org/10.1038/s41590-021-01122-w

[109] William A. Haseltine. Forbes. Aug 25, 2022. Solving the question of Covid variant increased fitness is like deciphering a Rubik;s cube. https://www.forbes. com/sites/williamhaseltine/2022/08/25/solving-the-question-of-covid-variant-increased-fitness-is-like-deciphering-a-rubiks-cube/?sh=389a403c6f56

CHAPTER 12

Long COVID Zombies

When there is no more room in hell, the dead will walk the earth.

—*Ken Foree*

The insistent ring of the alarm pierced through Sankari's slumber. She groaned as she rolled over, stretching out painfully to silence it. She lay there, hand outstretched toward the bedside table, half-awake, willing her body to move. It took Sankari all morning to get going these days. Her body felt as if it belonged to someone else, not really under her command. She could barely summon the will to do the most mundane of tasks. It wasn't that she was depressed. She wasn't, but her muscles seemed to have no strength. Ever since she'd had COVID four weeks ago, she hadn't been the same.

She coughed a dry hack as she slowly struggled into a sitting position on the edge of her bed. Her head felt dizzy and foggy, as if she had a hangover or she had taken too much Benadryl. Her husband had left for work long ago. She looked at the clock—11:30 a.m.!

One month ago, Sankari would have been up at 5:30 a.m. and at work by 7:00 a.m. By now, she'd have put in five hours of productive work at her marketing firm. But that seemed a lifetime away now. All that belonged to another person. A pre-COVID person. A person who was long gone, leaving behind this zombie, hollowed shell of a woman.

She felt neither alive nor dead, — stuck in some halfway hell, a purgatory of ennui.

Post-Acute Sequelae of COVID (PASC)

From the beginning, the media focused on the hospitalizations, the ICU bed occupancy, and the lonely deaths because the drama attracted the media. It was riveting video and print copy. But everyone ignored something that was very evident to us at the frontlines of primary care by the end of the first thirty days. My patients were not getting better even after they had cleared the virus. Two weeks post COVID infection, most of my patients would be testing negative for the virus by RT-PCR, yet they would tell me that they were not well.

For every hundred individuals who contracted the virus, only fifteen would become sick enough to require hospitalization. Out of those fifteen, five would require treatment in an ICU. Out of those five, three would die. But the eighty-five patients who never got sick enough to merit hospitalization faced an illness that continued to drag on for six to nine months, with no energy and a constellation of chronic symptoms. Some would not recover for twelve to eighteen months.

This feature of the pandemic was not appreciated by policymakers until much later. The impact of the pandemic on national productivity and on the available workforce was not a simple measure of the mortality rate. About 33 percent of people who got COVID were still unwell and unable to function at their pre-COVID level at six months after clearing the virus, regardless of the severity of their original disease. They called these people "long-haulers." Their condition was called "Long-COVID."

Eventually, academics would give this a formal name—post-acute sequelae of COVID (PASC)—but Long COVID was far more succinct and descriptive than this turgid academic phrase.[110] Researchers have

---

[110] H. E,. Davis, L. McCorkell, J. M. Vogel, et al., "Long COVID: Major Findings, Mechanisms and Recommendations," *Nat Rev Microbiol* (2023), https://doi.org/10.1038/s41579-022-00846-2.

yet to find the Occam's razor that offers a unified explanation of the bewildering array of presentations seen in Long COVID.[111]. Thus, Long COVID patients may present with evidence of one, some, or all the following organ system dysfunctions:

Heart—cardiac impairment, myocardial inflammation, POTS (a condition with palpitations on simple change of posture)

Lung—abnormal gas exchange

Immune system—autoimmunity, mast cell activation syndrome

Pancreas—diabetes, pancreatic injury

Gut—gut dysbiosis, viral persistence, and viral reservoir

Nervous system—dysautonomia, neuroinflammation, small fiber neuropathy, reduced blood flow, ME/CFS (encephalomyelitis / chronic fatigue syndrome)

Kidneys—renal damage

Blood vessels—abnormal clotting, micro-clots, stroke, DVT, pulmonary embolism, endothelial dysfunction, microangiopathy

Reproductive system—erectile dysfunction, reduced sperm count, menstrual problems

While the final picture and mechanism of pathogenesis is far from clear, there is increasing data pointing to a systemic dysregulation of whole-body inflammatory cascades resulting in multiple organ dysfunction on a long-term basis. Fatigue disproportionate to the level of exertion, chronic dry cough and shortness of breath, sleep disturbance, loss of concentration and memory recall and a general cognitive impairment described as brain fog, and heart palpitations are some of the most prevalent symptoms reported.

Indeed, there is tantalizing evidence that aspirin may be beneficial in the recovery from COVID. As early as April 2020, it was standard practice at my clinic to place all patients who were recovering from

---

[111] Occam's Razor—*lex parsimoniae* or the law of parsimony, attributed to William Occam, states that when faced with competing hypotheses about the same prediction, one should prefer the one with the fewest assumptions. Or in other words, the simplest explanation is usually the best one.

COVID and who were without contraindications to aspirin use, on extended low-dose aspirin therapy.[112]

One doctor colleague described Long COVID as a low-level smoldering fire that keeps burning the body long after the original inferno has died down. For us in the primary care trenches of health care this was the continuing challenge of SARS-CoV-2. It was not enough for us to stop the reaper from claiming our patients' souls. We had to wrest their bodies from his grasp. We had to bring them back from the dead.

In our clinic, we used every tool that could help—aspirin; vitamin D and vitamin C; zinc and magnesium; and well-recognized herbal anti-inflammatory human food-grade supplements like green-lipped mussel, devil's claw root extracts, Boswellia serrata (frankincense), cinnamon, black pepper, and turmeric. The criteria for which ones were recommended were based on only those with scientific literature

---

[112] Peter W. Horby, Guilherme Pessoa-Amorim, Natalie Staplin, Jonathan R. Emberson, Mark Campbell, Enti Spata, Leon Peto, Nigel J. Brunskill, Simon Tiberi, Victor Chew, Thomas Brown, Hasan Tahir, Beate Ebert, David Chadwick, Tony Whitehouse, Rahuldeb Sarkar, Clive Graham, J. Kenneth Baillie, Buddha Basnyat, Maya H. Buch, Lucy C. Chappell, Jeremy Day, Saul N. Faust, Raph L. Hamers, Thomas Jaki, Edmund Juszczak, Katie Jeffery, Wei Shen Lim, Alan Montgomery, Andrew Mumford, Kathryn Rowan, Guy Thwaites, Marion Mafham, Richard Haynes, and Martin J Landray, "Aspirin in Patients Admitted to Hospital with COVID-19 (RECOVERY): A Randomized, Controlled, Open Label, Platform Trial," RECOVERY Collaborative Group, *The Lancet* 339, no. 10,320: 143–51; Francesco Santoro, Ivan J. Núñez-Gil, Enrica Vitale, María C. Viana-Llamas, Rodolfo Romero, Charbel Maroun Eid, Gisela Feltes Guzman, Victor Manuel Becerra-Muñoz, Inmaculada Fernández Rozas, Aitor Uribarri, Emilio Alfonso-Rodriguez, Marcos García Aguado, Jia Huang, Alex Fernando Castro Mejía, Juan Fortunato Garcia Prieto, Javier Elola, Fabrizio Ugo, Enrico Cerrato, Jaime Signes-Costa, Sergio Raposeiras Roubin, Jorge Luis Jativa Mendez, Carolina Espejo Paeres, Alvaro López Masjuan, Francisco Marin, Federico Guerra, Ibrahim El-Battrawy, Bernardo Cortese, Harish Ramakrishna, Julian Perez-Villacastín, Antonio Fernandez-Ortiz, and Natale Daniele Brunetti, "Aspirin Therapy on Prophylactic Anticoagulation for Patients Hospitalized with COVID-19: A Propensity Score-Matched Cohort Analysis of the HOPE-COVID-19 Registry," *Journal of the American Heart Association* 11, no. 13, June 22, 2022.

supporting their effectiveness as exerting an anti-inflammatory effect at either the lab or clinical level. Some of the agents had ample evidence as inhibitors of pro-inflammatory cytokines like TNF-alfa, IL-6, COX2, and leukotrienes.[113] All of these could be purchased in capsule form on Amazon, and I would give my patients instruction sheets on how to take them after screening their records to eliminate potential conflicts with whatever other medicines they may be on. It was not a clinical trial. But all over the world, physicians like me were doing whatever they could with whatever they had using whatever judgement they could bring to bear to relieve the suffering of their patients. This was medicine being practiced in the heat and fog of battle with vigilance towards doing no harm in the hope of maximal good as we waited for science to catch up and provide us with validated and quantified tools.

The toll of COVID on the population cannot be measured simply based on lives lost or economic damage incurred. The immensity of loss will continue to reverberate in our societies for generations. What is the measure of the lost education of children shut out from in-person learning for 2 years? How shall we quantify the stunting of psychological development of adolescents locked in quarantine? What happens to the future of children who lose one or both parents to disease? What is the cost to society of families pushed below the poverty line due to the

---

[113] T. Brendler, "From Bush Medicine to Modern Phytopharmaceutical: A Bibliographic Review of Devil's Claw (Harpagophytum spp.)," *Pharmaceuticals* 14 (2021), 726; H. Safayhi, E. R. Sailer, and H. P. Ammon, "Mechanism of 5-LIPOXYGENASE INHIBITION by acetyl-11-Keto-Beta-Boswellic Acid," *Mol Pharmacol* 47, no. 6 (June 1995): 1,212–6, PMID: 7603462; H. P. Ammon, H. Safayhi, T. Mack, and J. Sabieraj, "Mechanism of Anti-Inflammatory Actions of Curcumine and Boswellic Acids," *J Ethnopharmacol* 38, no. 2–3 (March 1993): 113–9, doi: 10.1016/0378-8741(93)90005-p, PMID: 8510458; S. Brien, P. Prescott, B. Coghlan, N. Bashir, and G. Lewith, "Systematic Review of the Nutritional Supplement Perna Canaliculus (Green-Lipped Mussel) in the Treatment of Osteoarthritis," *QJM* 101, no. 3 (March 2008): 167–79, doi: 10.1093/qjmed/hcm108, epub January 25, 2008, PMID: 18222988; and M. Z. Siddiqui, "Boswellia Serrata, a Potential Anti-Inflammatory Agent: An Overview," *Indian J Pharm Sci* 73, no. 3 (May 2011): 255–61, doi: 10.4103/0250-474X.93507, PMID: 22457547, PMCID: PMC3309643.

death of income generating adults? Who measures the lingering impact of orphaned children swallowed by the predation of human trafficking? How do you measure the family that must manage without a parent who is incapacitated due to Long COVID? When a parent dies, the survivors bury them and move on. There is closure and a new beginning. But Long COVID is a continuing funeral with no end. In this, the limitations of conventional health care become glaringly evident. Physicians are simply not trained to handle anything beyond an interventional approach to health. Most physicians are woefully unprepared to educate patients in lifestyle and behavioral transformation. If they can't have a drug or a procedure to prescribe, they are lost before the litany of complaints of their Long COVID patients. But there is some light at the end of this tunnel. Recent data show a reduction in the number of long COVID cases nationally. Much of this is attributed to the prevalence of vaccination and the development of the beginnings of herd immunity. And this is ultimately the greatest vindication for the pro-vaccination argument that one can find.

CHAPTER 13

A New Normal

We sense that "normal" isn't coming back, that we are being born into a new normal: a new kind of society, a new relationship to the earth, a new experience of being human.
—*Charles Eisenstein*

I pulled up into my parking slot in front of the clinic. I no longer see as many COVID-positive patients, and those that I do see have mild cases. Their symptoms are seldom greater in intensity than those of the seasonal flu. Every now and then, one of my patients develops pneumonia, though that is becoming rarer these days. Still, for my patients with concomitant heart disease, heart failure, or kidney disease, COVID remains a lethal disease. In this, it is behaving like any other viral illness.

Yet, in many ways, life for all of us has changed irrevocably. Masking in health-care facilities has become a new normal, and that is unlikely to change any time soon. I do believe the world is beginning to comprehend that we exist in a precarious balance with the environment and that this fragile balance is indeed becoming more unstable. The pandemic has made everyone take a hard look at what they are working for, what they are working toward, and for whom and why.

The great pandemic was accompanied by the great die-off and followed by the great resignation. There is something about coming face-to-face with your own mortality that wakes you out of the torpor of sameness that ruled before November 2019. The lockdown and isolation of 2020 and 2021 has made us all value the small things. I, for one, take great pleasure in sitting three feet across from my wife and sipping coffee face-to-face, maskless. Gatherings, small and large, feel so much more precious now.

At work, 25 percent of my billable service is now accomplished by a video chat in a tele-visit. Insurers keep threatening to stop paying for it, but the market has adopted it. It is now the new normal for health-care services, and I seriously doubt it will be dropped. Last November I hired a data analyst at my clinic. He works remotely from home three days and in the office two days in one week and then remotely two days and in the office three days in the next week. Globally, industry has accepted the concept of teleworking and found that productivity has even gone up.

One thing that I truly miss about the pandemic is the surge in wildlife that I saw in April, May, and June 2020 during the height of the lockdowns. Roads were wide open, with zero traffic; the air became clear and smog-free; and the mountains were visible. Crystal clear from my window, I could see foxes, raccoons and deer playing boldly in my front lawn. While all humanity was choking and gasping for breath, nature and wildlife were taking a huge breath of fresh air and discovering a new freedom. It was impossible not to be struck by the irony and poetic justice of it all.

Still, I am aware that a sword hangs by a thread above us. These two years were a warning to humankind and to me. The reaper has not gone. He has merely sat back on a reclining chair, and he is watching us all with his toothy grin. He has myriad reasons to return. The environment is full of animals carrying still unknown viruses and microbes' humankind has never seen.

As recent as February 10, 2023, The Guardian reported the finding of four seals dead on the Scottish coastline infected with the H5N1 strain of bird flu.[114] Professor Ursula Hofle of the University of Castilla,

---

[114] Phoebe Weston. The Guardian. Feb 10, 2023. Four dead seals test positive for bird flu in Scotland. https://www.theguardian.com/world/2023/feb/10/four-dead-seals-test-positive-bird-flu-scotland-aoe

in comments about bird flu transmission, admitted, "There's definitely increasing evidence for bird to mammal and mammal to mammal transmission."

Countries everywhere are beginning to take a hard look at pandemic preparedness. Separately, our intoxication with our intellectual prowess continues to seduce us with the illusion that we have all the answers and that we can engineer the outcome of our species at will. Governments are beefing up their biosecurity and biosafety preparedness. Organizations and scientists are waking up to the fact that, while research is necessary, the level of transparency and oversight also must significantly increase to ensure that our science does not run amuck and become our own executioner.

Our own rapacious appetite for consumption continues to invade forbidden domains through deforestation and ecological degradation. Climate change is no longer a future event; it is here among us now! It will continue to push us toward chaos and strain our already meager resources for controlling our environment to our convenience. Our world is changing and not always for the better. Governments are taking steps to be better prepared.[115]

Vaccine development is sorely needed, and there is a greater urgency now behind their development. Equally necessary is a global education campaign to confront anti-vax and vaccine hesitancy conversations that are crippling even the best public health effort. Supply chain redundancy needs to be built into economies. Certain critical items need to be stockpiled or manufacturing must be accomplished in a disaster-resilient model. I believe that ordinary citizens will need to keep a stock of sanitation supplies and necessities to serve as a buffer for unexpected supply chain shortages.

The pandemic lay bare the total collapse of the US public health system for the world to see. We are woefully ill-equipped in the areas of epidemiology, testing, and contact tracing. The poorest African nation

---

[115] Dennis Normille. Science. Feb 9, 2023. Japan moves top bolster vaccine R&D after Covid-19 exposed startling weakness. https://www.science.org/content/article/japan-moves-bolster-vaccine-r-d-after-covid-19-exposed-startling-weakness

has a better corps of public health workers than the United States. The US health-care system runs on a business model of intervention, not prevention. The kind of problems that will emerge for us are better handled on a preventive basis. This will require a significant transformational shift of an entire industry.

In addition, the study of infectious disease is never more necessary than now. But the pandemic put on display how the world treated Dr. Anthony Fauci, the country and the world's foremost infectious disease expert.[116] In 2022, a full 44 percent of infectious disease fellowship programs went begging for candidates.[117] Paul Pottinger, director of the infectious disease training program at the University of Washington, speaks of the "denigration of people who speak the truth," noting people may be tired of being beaten up on.

The pandemic, for a brief, searing twenty-four-month period, ripped off the scab over the festering wounds of modern human society and has revealed the huge inequities and gaps we have as people. These gaps are not deficiencies but, rather, serious failings that, if not corrected, will destroy us all.

In November 2021, Dr. Fauci spoke at the STAT Summit, a gathering of the world's foremost experts in the fields of biotech, pharma, policy, health tech, and business on the challenges facing us all. "How do you change a mindset in a country that is completely antithetical to a response to an outbreak? If ever there was any phenomenon that required people pulling together in a society, it's an outbreak that's killing hundreds of thousands of people. I don't know how we're going to get that divisiveness behind us," he said.[118]

---

[116] Andrew Joseph. Stat. Nov 15, 2022. 'I pushed back': Fauci on how his response to Trump on Covid turned him into 'public enemy No. 1' https://www.statnews.com/2022/11/15/fauci-on-how-he-became-public-enemy-no-1/

[117] Andrew Joseph. Stat. Dec 7, 2022.Limits of 'Fauci effect': infectious disease applicants plummet, and hospitals are scrambling. https://www.statnews.com/2022/12/07/infectious-disease-fellowship-drop-in-applicants/

[118] Andrew Joseph. Stat. Nov 16, 2021. Fauci on next phase of the Covid-19 pandemic and the 'insanity' of the threats he faces pushing for masks, vaccines. https://www.statnews.com/2021/11/16/fauci-interview-insanity-covid-stat-summit/

The Poverty Mindset

The pandemic's ugliest face was the idea of "us versus them" that is pervasive in us all. I call this the "poverty mindset." Years ago, I had given a talk on the mindset of success, and I spoke of this as the "not enough life." I said that 99 percent of people all over the world live their lives as if there is a perpetual shortage of resources. We live as if there is "not enough" of the things that matter to us, the things we want or need—not enough time, not enough space, not enough money, not enough friends, not enough love, not enough recognition, not enough, not enough, not enough. I called this the poverty mindset because the "not enough life" is a poverty that can never be filled. You don't have to be poor to have the poverty mindset. Some extremely wealthy and successful individuals live lives trapped in this thinking.

The worldview of this mindset is based on treating resources as if they are mere physical objects limited by boundaries of space and time. So, to survive, compete, and win, we humans must grab and snatch and claw these resources, snatch them out of our fellow's mouth, if necessary, before they are gone — taken by someone else or some other thing. We do this in the name of courage, competitiveness, and success and in the name of some of our highest attributes. The pandemic unveiled the darkness of this not enough mentality on a global level.

But the mentality of poverty is completely reversed if we recognize that the ultimate resource, we possess is not the resources themselves but the relationships between them—the interconnectedness of us all. "Truly successful people, high performance people, do not operate on the mentality that resources are finite," I said. "They operate on the principle that their primary resource is the relationships of the things they have power over. This is their real asset. The interconnectedness of their network. They grow by expanding the reach of their network. The health of these relationships is the only resource that they are concerned with. They move from living in the poverty mindset to living in the abundance mindset. They move from being hoarders and consumers to being stewards of their lives and of their world. Successful people with an abundance mindset are like a rising tide. They lift all boats."

The pandemic revealed this interconnectedness of us all in a way as never before. Whether it was the spread of a single virion particle from China to Alaska or the fact that the paper we wipe our bottoms with is dependent on the health of a Far East Asian worker or the fact that our atmosphere and our wilderness is connected to our use of this planet, the pandemic showed that rather than us versus them, we had better begin thinking of us and them as we.

Will we learn? Will we remember? Will you?

EPILOGUE

At the edge of a clearing in the Brazilian rainforest, a bulldozer topples a tall tree. The giant tree hits the ground in slow motion like a Goliath of a bygone age struck down by a diminutive, tool-bearing David. The crash of timber barely drowns the indignant screeching protest of howler monkeys and birds at this destruction of their home. There is a rent in the canopy where the tree stood, and the dozer operator can see the purple twilight of the evening sky silhouetting the swarm of bats disturbed by the fall of the giant. The operator shuts off the dozer engine and climbs down the ladder. Time to call it a day, he thinks as he walks over to the campsite.

A bat swoops past his head. Something wet and slimy plops on his shoulder, and he wipes it. "Ugh! Bat shit." He grunts as he wipes his wet excrement covered right hand on a branch. He sits down by the campfire and reaches across to pour a cup of coffee. Reaching into his backpack, he fishes out a pack of Marlboros and strikes a light. The cigarette glows between the fingers of his right hand as he inhales a satisfying lungful. His lips moisten the paper of the cigarette as it rests between his still slightly wet fingers. He draws deeply, and the tobacco vapor, smoke, water vapor, and a few molecules of bat excrement swoosh into the warm humid passages of his lungs. In the distance, a shrill screech of a howler monkey fills the night air as radiant full moon floats out of a cloud in the sky.

ABOUT THE AUTHOR

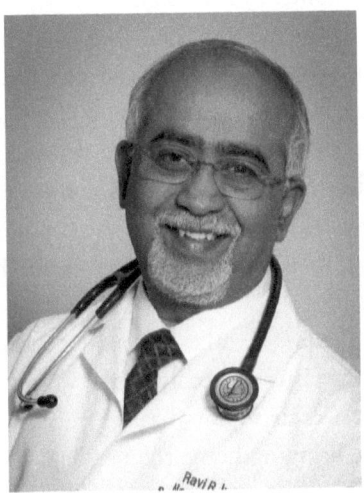

Photo Credit: AJ Photoz

Acclaimed as 2024's fastest rising speaker and expert on People First Leadership and recognized in the same company as Simon Sinek, and Pete Burbridge of the Dale Carnegie Institute in the space of thought leaders and pioneers, Dr Ravi Iyer, MD operates in the space of blending high performance teams, and profitability with exceptionally high levels of employee satisfaction and customer service.

A physician-scientist, inventor, author, short film actor, transdisciplinary polymath and entrepreneur with research publications in the mechanisms of gene controls and several patents on human and veterinary medicines and devices, Dr Iyer's professional accomplishments include over 40 years of experience spanning the fields of science, medicine, biochemistry, molecular biology, and pharmaceuticals, a 9-year Directorship of a Hospice caring for dying patients, and a 4-year Chairmanship of a 225-bed hospital. His contributions have been recognized worldwide by organizations such as Marqui's Who's Who in America and Who's Who in TOP Doctors of America.

His extensive background of over 40 years in the fields of medicine, science, basic research, drug regulation, and vaccine development and creating and leading high-performance teams puts him in a unique position to speak about the issues of human health and wellness, leadership and human potential development with insight, clarity, incisive depth, and deep compassion about the human condition.

Dr. Iyer is a sought-after speaker and coach at public and media events and his Workshop on Leadership & Living has been rated as transformational for enabling individuals, teams and organizations to discover their grounding narrative and showing them the methods by which they can remain connected with that space, thereby allowing them immense focus and creativity as well as resilience and flexibility in navigating the uncertainties of their life.

In The Reaper's Dance, he takes the reader into the frontlines of the global battle against the virus and analyzes the various forces and decisions that unleashed the most catastrophic disaster humankind has experienced in this century, while bringing home the personal horror, pain, struggles, and triumphs of the common people who ultimately faced and fought the disease of their times. In a fast-flowing style of writing, Dr. Iyer takes the reader from the clinic into the homes of COVID patients and into the science that may have unleashed the horror, as well as the science that created the redemption from it in a book that grips you from the first word to its haunting end.

He is currently working on his next books and his work may be found at: www.driyer.com

www.ingramcontent.com/pod-product-compliance
Lightning Source LLC
Chambersburg PA
CBHW030938240526
45463CB00015B/405